Feeding and Swallowing Disorders in Dementia

Feeding and Swallowing Disorders in Dementia

Jacqueline Kindell

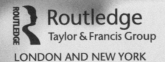

Routledge
Taylor & Francis Group

LONDON AND NEW YORK

First published 2002 by Speechmark Publishing Ltd.

Published 2017 by Routledge
2 Park Square, Milton Park, Abingdon, Oxon OX14 4RN
711 Third Avenue, New York, NY 10017, USA

Routledge is an imprint of the Taylor & Francis group, an informa business

British Library Cataloguing in Publication Data

Kindell, Jacqueline
    Feeding and swallowing disorders in dementia
    1. Dementia – Patients – Diseases   2. Ingestion disorders
    3. Dementia – Patients – Care
    I. Title
    616.8'3

ISBN: 9780863883125 (pbk)

Contents

Tables

Acknowledgements

The author is especially grateful to Mariani Tanton, Barbara Tanner, Tessa Pemberton, Hilary Curtis and Astrid Cameron, who undertook the initial stages of this work.

Thanks are also due to members of the Northern UK Speech and Language Therapy Special Interest Group in Old Age Psychiatry, Hilary Smith (Specialist Speech and Language Therapist), and Dr RC Baldwin (Consultant Psychiatrist for the Elderly), who have given me help and provided valuable feedback on this project.

About the Author

Jacqueline Kindell is a specialist speech and language therapist, who has worked in Old Age Psychiatry in Manchester since 1992. During this time Jacqueline has worked as part of a specialist multi-disciplinary team, providing assessment, treatment and management advice to people with dementia and their carers. A significant part of this role has been working with people who experience feeding and swallowing difficulties. Jacqueline is secretary of the Northern Speech and Language Therapy Special Interest Group in Old Age Psychiatry, and is a member of the 'Expert Group for Mental Health' for the Royal College of Speech and Language Therapists' Clinical Guidelines Project. She has recently moved to a new post as a speech and language therapist and Therapy Services Manager in Old Age Psychiatry at Stockport NHS Trust.

Introduction

Dementia is a syndrome that involves chronic or progressive disturbance of multiple cognitive functions, emotional control and social behaviour in clear consciousness (*International Classification of Diseases*, ICD-10). This leads to increasing difficulty in carrying out activities of daily living.

Carers and staff working with individuals with dementia will be aware of the range of problems presented at meal times, and the challenge these difficulties present in terms of management. There is an increasing body of literature documenting such difficulties, highlighting both feeding and swallowing disorders, and possible strategies to manage these problems.

Weight loss in individuals with dementia, particularly Alzheimer's disease, is well recognised although debate continues as to the reason for this. Guyonnet *et al* (1998) studied weight loss in 76 people with slight to moderate Alzheimer's disease living in the community. Results showed that 44.2 per cent of subjects showed a weight loss greater than 4 per cent in one year. They advise that, given the significance of the problem, regular monitoring of nutritional status should occur as soon as a diagnosis of dementia is given.

Singh *et al* (1988) asked 'why are Alzheimer's patients thin?'. They examined 74 hospitalised patients, and found that those with Alzheimer's weighed less than those with multi-infarct dementia, and less than non-demented elderly controls. However, the reason for the weight loss remained uncertain. A number of theories have been outlined in the literature, including difficulty feeding, increased activity, changes in appetite, changes in taste and sensation, and metabolic disturbance. Du *et al* (1993) asked whether weight loss is a core symptom of Alzheimer's disease, reflecting specific regional brain damage, or a secondary consequence of the dementia. It seems likely that there are a variety of reasons for loss of weight, in people with dementia. This is due to differences in the type of dementia, the stage of the disease, and individual differences in physical and mental state. It should also be noted that some people with dementia have been reported to overeat. This problem, called 'hyperphagia', seems to occur at some stage in about a quarter of people with dementia (Trinkle, 1992), further highlighting the variability present. Some nutritional deficiency disorders may give rise to treatable causes of dementia – for example deficiency of vitamin B_{12}, folic acid, thiamine and nicotinic acid. Though such causes of dementia are relatively small in number, they are important because they are potentially reversible (Burns, 1995).

There is a great deal of evidence that people in residential care, particularly individuals with dementia, experience increasing difficulty feeding themselves. Siebens et al (1986) studied 240 residents in a nursing facility and found that only 53 per cent were totally independent eaters. Those who were dependent needed assistance ranging from verbal supervision to physical assistance (32 per cent of cases). Eating dependency did not correlate with age, but with a variety of factors including impaired cognition. Volicer et al (1989) found that in a sample of 73 institutionalised individuals with Alzheimer's disease, 50 per cent needed at least some feeding assistance and 32 per cent had swallowing difficulties. Using a screening tool, Steele et al (1997) studied mealtimes in 349 residents in a home for the aged. She found that 87 per cent of the individuals showed mealtime difficulties. Sixty-eight per cent had signs of swallowing dysfunction; 46 per cent had poor oral intake; 40 per cent exhibited challenging behaviours, and 35 per cent had positioning problems. Du et al (1993) followed up 81 people with Alzheimer's disease, and found a significant link between ability to eat independently and weight loss: as their ability to feed themselves decreased, so generally did their weight.

The inability to eat puts such individuals at risk of malnutrition. This in turn increases vulnerability to infection, and to other conditions that contribute to increased morbidity and mortality. Sandman et al (1987) studied 44 severely demented, institutionalised individuals, and found that those who were malnourished had four times as many infectious periods treated by antibiotics as those with no malnutrition. Rudman and Feller (1989) have highlighted how poor nutrition can contribute to a cycle of difficulty in fighting infection. Ek et al (1990) reported that, in elderly hospital patients, malnutrition leads to such complications as higher frequency of pressure sores, delayed wound healing and higher mortality rates, than in those with adequate nutritional status.

Difficulty with swallowing often leads to reduced oral intake, and puts people at risk of aspiration of food particles into the lungs, leading in some cases to aspiration pneumonia (Logemann, 1983). Feinberg et al (1992) found, in a retrospective videofluoroscopy study of 131 individuals with advanced dementia, that only 7 per cent showed a normal swallow. Hudson *et al* (2000), in a review article, highlighted the interdependent relationship between malnutrition and swallowing difficulty. Swallowing problems lead to nutritional decline, and equally malnutrition may increase the risk and severity of aspiration episodes, due to reduced respiratory muscle strength and impaired immune function. Siebens *et al* (1986) concluded that eating dependency is associated with multiple impairments and early mortality.

In a longitudinal study of 79 people with dementia in long-term care, Wang *et al* (1998) found that weight loss is not necessarily unremitting during institutionalisation. They argue that when resources are directed to nutritional aspects of care, then nursing, dietary, therapy and physician staff are able to maintain an individual's weight and survival for extended periods, even in very impaired residents. VOICES (1998) gave nutritional guidelines for food prepared for people with dementia in residential or nursing homes, and provided some very helpful information regarding eating and swallowing problems in this population. The Alzheimer's Society of Great Britain (2000), in their report *Food for Thought,* found many respondents to their survey felt that people with dementia were not given enough to eat and drink in hospitals and care homes. They also felt that an individual's needs and difficulties were often not recognised, and that there was a lack of choice, and a lack of time on the part of staff to provide assistance with eating. The Society produced a number of key recommendations and concrete advice.

It is the responsibility of staff looking after people with dementia to identify and manage these problems as best they can. The above studies have highlighted a variety of factors that need to be examined when difficulty with eating arises. When people can no longer feed themselves, others must take over this task. The individual becomes reliant for their eating on the skill and motivation of others (Kolodny & Malek, 1991). This can be a staff- and time-intensive process. For example, it has been estimated that the cost of managing eating dependency may account for 25 per cent of the total cost of caring for nursing home residents (Zimmer, 1975). In some instances, despite dedicated staff, inappropriate or at times dangerous feeding techniques are used, because such individuals lack the knowledge or training required (Kolodny & Malek, 1991). Therefore it is also important that the practices used by staff at mealtimes are examined. Assessment and management of eating, feeding and swallowing involves all members of the multi-disciplinary team – doctors, nurses, support staff, occupational therapists, speech and language therapists, dietitians and physiotherapists, along with catering staff and managers. Relatives are also vital to this process. It is the role of the speech and language therapist to provide a detailed description of the swallowing problem and associated factors that influence eating. Following on from this, management involves instigating strategies to reduce difficulties, maintain skills, educate staff and relatives, and identify individuals who need further assessment by other disciplines.

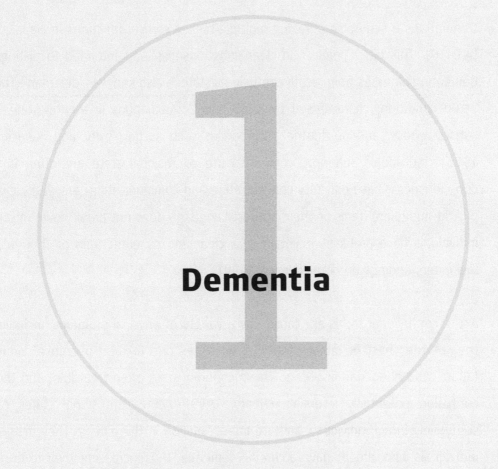

Dementia

Differential diagnosis of dementia and acute confusional state

Dementia is a syndrome affecting multiple higher cortical functions in clear consciousness (ICD-10). This latter point – 'in clear consciousness' – is intended to distinguish chronic dementing illnesses from 'acute confusional states', also know as 'delerium'. The latter is an acute condition, characterised by rapid onset; fluctuations in mental state; clouding of consciousness, and psychiatric disturbances such as perplexity and hallucinosis (Burns, 1995). Individuals suffering from an acute confusional state are often in and out of consciousness; have difficulty concentrating and communicating; are easily distracted, and pick at imaginary items or their clothes. Language does not break down into aphasia, but individuals have problems maintaining a clear and coherent train of thought, and verbal misunderstandings do occur (Neary, 1999).

Acute confusional states are caused by a variety of physical problems, including infections (eg, of the chest or urinary tract); toxic states due to drug overdose; kidney and liver failure, and endocrine disorders. These conditions are often treatable, and the associated confusion potentially reversible (Neary, 1999). Acute confusional states can occur in cognitively intact individuals and are more common in the elderly. They may also occur in individuals who already have a chronic dementia, thus increasing their level of confusion. This is often referred to as an 'acute on chronic state'. Treatment can be given, and the acute confusional state may lift, revealing again the underlying chronic state.

Dementia and changes in eating

Turning to chronic or progressive dementia, it is important to remember that dementia is not a disease in itself, but a syndrome, caused by a variety of diseases of the brain. In recent years there has been growing interest in the way different dementing diseases affect the brain. Neary (1999) states that different cerebral diseases tend to affect certain brain regions and spare others. Because cognitive processes (eg, memory, language, praxis, perception, spatial function and executive skills) are organised regionally in the brain, different diseases are associated with different patterns of cognitive impairment. This theory moves away from the traditional view that dementia is a global deterioration of function and considers the 'cognitive features' of dementia. In addition, there has been increased interest in the psychiatric and behavioural symptoms of dementia including depression, hallucinations, delusions, aggression, agitation, pacing and eating disorders. Such behaviours are often termed 'noncognitive features', or 'behavioural and psychological symptoms of dementia (BPSD)'. (See Purandare *et al*, 2000 for a review of this area.) Such problems cause significant stress, for both the sufferer and the carer.

There is very little research available on the different patterns of eating, feeding and swallowing impairments in different types of dementia. Both cognitive and noncognitive features can impact on eating skills. Tables 1.1 and 1.2 illustrate some of the difficulties presented. These are explained further in Chapter 3. Physical and neurological changes also

TABLE 1.1 **COGNITIVE FEATURES THAT IMPACT ON EATING SKILLS**

Cognitive difficulty	Effect on eating
Memory disturbance	Forgetting when last ate Forgetting when next meal will be Losing track of the task of eating
Perceptual and spatial difficulties	Difficulty locating crockery, cutlery and food Difficulty recognising food and utensils
Apraxia (limb and oral apraxia)	Difficulty using a knife and fork Difficulty performing voluntary actions, such as opening the mouth to a spoon or moving food from the front to the back of the mouth
Language difficulties	Difficulty expressing food preferences Problems understanding mealtime instructions
Executive (also termed frontal lobe) dysfunction	Socially inappropriate mealtime behaviour Eating too quickly Cramming food Altered food choice

TABLE 1.2 **NONCOGNITIVE FEATURES THAT IMPACT ON EATING SKILLS**

Noncognitive difficulty	Effect on eating
Pacing/agitation	Problems sitting at the table Poor concentration on eating Increased energy requirements
Aggression	Difficulty accepting help from others Refusal to eat/be fed/sit at the table Throwing food or hitting out at the feeder
Depression	Poor appetite and food refusals, often leading to associated weight loss Slow eating
Delusions	Food refusals due to delusional ideas about food or those serving it – eg, that it is poison
Hallucinations	Disturbance in concentration at mealtimes due to hallucinations – eg, 'seeing' flies on the table

occur in different degrees and stages in the different types of dementia, for example weakness, incoordination, rigidity and difficulty with initiating of movement, as well as loss of sensory functions. These can have the profound effect on both feeding and swallowing seen in other populations, such as stroke victims and those suffering from Parkinson's disease.

Alzheimer's disease

Disturbance in memory is usually the earliest symptom of Alzheimer's disease, causing the person to have difficulty remembering recent events. Individuals may also have problems with 'immediate memory', causing them to lose track of what they are doing, or the thread of the conversation (Snowden, 1999). However, Alzheimer's is not just a disorder of memory, but also leads to problems with language skills; recognition of objects and faces (perception); locating and orientating objects in space (spatial skills), and carrying out patterns of movement such as dressing (praxis). Also associated are disorders of mood, delusions, hallucinations and behavioural problems such as aggression, wandering and sleep disturbance (Burns, *et al*, 1995). This constellation of features is often referred to as the '5 As' of Alzheimer's disease:

◆ Amnesia

◆ Aphasia

◆ Agnosia

◆ Apraxia

◆ Associated (noncognitive features) (Burns *et al*, 1995).

This leads to increasing difficulty in carrying out even simple activities of daily living. Physical signs are usually absent until the later stages of the illness, and consist of akinesia, rigidity and myoclonus (sudden contraction of the muscles), due to involvement of the subcortical structures (Neary, 1999). In the very late stages, postural problems occur, and may be so severe that the body becomes flexed, with the person lying curled up (Leeds, 1960).

In the author's experience, individuals usually have declining skills in self-feeding in the mild and moderate stages of the illness, due to limb apraxia and spatial disturbance which, ultimately in the later stages, means that they have to be fed by others. In the early stages of the illness, changes in the swallowing mechanism have been reported (eg, Priefer, 1997); however, clinically swallowing problems are rarely a concern. It is in the later stages, when the person is fed by others, that significant swallowing problems emerge. Common problems begin with oral-stage difficulties – eg, overchewing, or holding food, followed later by more obvious delay in initiating a swallow, with pharyngeal difficulties and risk of aspiration. In some individuals, signs of oral apraxia can be clearly observed – eg, difficulty opening the mouth to a spoon when required, or within the oral stage of the swallow. In those with severe myoclonus, twitching can occur in the oral musculature, which can sometimes interfere with eating. Therefore swallowing problems in this population are not solely due to behavioural or cognitive deficits. There are physical and neurological changes, for example, in subcortical structures as described, that may impact on swallowing function.

Vascular (multi-infarct) dementia

Recurrent cortical strokes lead to increasing neurological and cognitive difficulties. Onset may be abrupt, and the progression stepwise as each stroke occurs. The difficulties presented depend on where in the brain damage has occurred, eg, aphasia, amnesia, etc. Neurological signs may include limb weakness, dysarthria of varying degrees, and swallowing difficulties. When small strokes occur in the subcortex, difficulties may be less obvious initially, and progression may not be as stepwise, but the accumulated damage gradually leads to slowness and rigidity in thinking, forgetfulness and problems in planning and sequencing mental events (Neary, 1999). In some individuals, strokes may occur in both the cortex and subcortex. Depression and emotional lability are particularly associated with vascular dementia (Burns *et al*, 1995).

People with vascular dementia can potentially have swallowing problems at any stage of the illness, due to stroke damage to the areas of the brain involved in swallowing. Such individuals are common on a speech and language therapy general medical caseload. In contrast to Alzheimer's disease, these individuals are more likely to be able to self-feed, yet have significant swallowing problems. As the dementia progresses, and more strokes occur, the more likely people are to develop swallowing problems.

Dementia of the Lewy body type

Dementia of the Lewy body type is increasingly becoming recognised. The condition is associated with Parkinson's disease, in which cell changes called 'Lewy bodies' are found in the cells in the brainstem. In dementia of the Lewy body type, however, Lewy bodies are found in cells outside the brainstem, in the cortex and subcortex (Neary, 1999).

McKeith *et al* (1996) outline criteria for this condition as:

1   Progressive cognitive decline that interferes with normal social or occupational function. Prominent or persistent memory impairment may not necessarily occur in the early stage, but is usually evident with progression. Deficits on tests of attention and of frontal-subcortical skills and visuospatial ability may be especially prominent.

2   Two of the following are essential for a diagnosis of probable Lewy body dementia:
     (a) Fluctuating cognition with pronounced variations in attention and alertness
     (b) Recurrent visual hallucinations that are typically well formed and detailed
     (c) Spontaneous motor features of Parkinsonism.

3   Features supportive of the diagnosis are:

   (a) Repeated falls

   (b) Syncope

   (c) Transient loss of consciousness

   (d) Neuroleptic (antipsychotic) sensitivity

   (e) Systemised delusions

   (f) Hallucinations in other modalities.

4   A diagnosis of Lewy body dementia is less likely in the presence of:

   (a) Stroke disease, evident as focal neurologic signs or on brain imaging

   (b) Evidence on physical examination and investigation, of any physical illness or other brain disorder, sufficient to account for the clinical picture.

In the author's experience, the feeding and swallowing problems of this group may vary along with their overall variability. Attentional problems may lead to distractibility at meal times, and the visuospatial difficulties may lead to problems in self-feeding. Those with significant Parkinsonian symptoms may have swallowing problems within the oral/pharyngeal stages (see Chapter 4), similar to those seen in Parkinson's disease.

Frontotemporal dementia (Pick's disease)

In Frontotemporal dementia, there is damage to the frontal and temporal lobes, leading to insidious and gradual change in personality and behaviour. It is associated with early decline in social interpersonal conduct; decline in manners and social graces, and antisocial and disinhibited behaviour. There is impaired regulation of personal conduct, leading to either inertia or overactivity, with emotional blunting and loss of insight. Other features may include mental rigidity; perseveration; stereotyped behaviour; echolalia, hyperorality and dietary changes (Neary *et al*, 1998). In contrast, memory and in particular spatial skills, are relatively well preserved. The condition usually has a presenile onset.

There is very little information on the eating, and especially swallowing problems, of this group. Neary *et al* (1999) and Bathgate *et al* (2001) have indicated that such individuals may initially lose the social graces associated with eating, and eat quickly, cramming food, and develop a likening for sweet foods. The cramming may be associated with coughing or choking on food. Because such individuals do not have spatial problems, they are often able to feed themselves later into the condition than those with Alzheimer's disease. The author has noted swallowing problems in clients with frontotemporal dementia, involving oral-stage difficulties with solid food at first, moving on to difficulties initiating a swallow on a variety of textures, together with risk of aspiration. This tends to occur in the later stages of the illness.

2

Production and Use
of this Resource Pack

An individual with no difficulty in feeding and swallowing has the ability to do the following:

◆ Recognise when they are hungry/thirsty

◆ Remember when they last ate, and plan when to eat next

◆ Seek out food, and recognise what is edible, and what is not

◆ Prepare food, so it is in an acceptable form to eat

◆ Use cutlery or their hands in a socially appropriate fashion to eat

◆ Judge how much to put in their mouth at once

◆ Judge an appropriate speed to eat

◆ Concentrate, and remember to continue with the task in hand (ignoring other distractions)

◆ Taste, and recognise, a variety of flavours and foods

◆ Chew effectively

◆ Elicit a co-ordinated swallow

◆ Direct material into the oesophagus, protecting the airway, with all textures

◆ Judge when they are full, and so when to stop eating.

Clearly, eating involves a range of functions including motor, sensory and cognitive skills. It also has significance in terms of cultural and social factors, as well as varying according to individual habits (Beck, 1981).

Kayser-Jones (1996) argues that eating habits of elderly people in nursing homes are highly individualised, and eating problems often occur due to a complex constellation of interacting factors, such as poor oral health, medication, clinical conditions, and lack of attention to individual food likes and dislikes. She highlights the importance of individualised care at mealtimes, observing that there is often a lack of ethnic food, unrecognised dysphagia and lack of attention to poor oral health, as well as a lack of assistance at mealtimes. Sidenvall and Ek (1993) found that problems with eating and nutritional deficits may be missed as part of the nursing assessment in hospital, and argue that, when recognised, eating dependency could be prevented. There is clearly a need to develop more proactive assessment and management of mealtime difficulties for these individuals. Watson (1997) discusses the difficulties surrounding this area, and suggests that further research is required, in particular into management strategies and measuring their effectiveness. For example, he argues that some of what we intuitively believe to be of benefit still requires investigation.

A basic version of this resource pack was developed by a group of speech and language therapists from the United Kingdom Northern Special Interest Group in Old Age Psychiatry, who worked with patients with dementia.

Members of the group were involved routinely with assessing and managing swallowing, and mealtime difficulties in individuals with dementia. It was recognised that the difficulties presented were often complex and variable, involving a range of skills. Difficulties varied between individuals, depending on the stage of their dementia, the type of dementia, co-occurring physical and sensory impairment, and differences in behaviour and personality. In addition, the wider eating environment impacted on the person's abilities, including the way staff fed and interacted with the individual.

The group felt that standard dysphagia (swallowing) assessments alone were too narrow to be used with this client group, because of the co-occurring problems with feeding (by both self and others) and behaviour. In addition, many individuals are unable to cooperate with such a process. Therefore, it was felt that a detailed tool was required to supplement such assessments, to highlight a range of possible mealtime difficulties for a given individual, and ways to manage these. Because most individuals referred were not 'nil by mouth', but still eating, information could be gathered most productively by using structured observation at mealtimes, as well as considering the history and presentation of the problem. Assessment and management of such difficulties requires a problem-solving approach, and this resource pack is designed to aid the process.

The group therefore produced a descriptive assessment as a way of meeting this need. They used cases from their own clinical practice to come to a consensus regarding the most commonly occurring mealtime difficulties, and successful ways to manage each problem area in clinical practice. The information was collated to form an assessment and management tool, which the author piloted on 18 people in hospital diagnosed by an old-age psychiatrist as suffering from dementia. Nine patients were consecutive referrals to speech and language therapy for assessment, and a further nine were identified by staff as having difficulty with feeding or swallowing. All were observed at mealtimes (in most cases on more than one occasion). Individual details are shown in Table 2.1.

TABLE 2.1 **DETAILS OF INDIVIDUALS OBSERVED IN THE PILOT STUDY**

Type of dementia	Number	Mini-mental state examination score	Ages
Vascular dementia	9	0–24	65–79
Alzheimer's disease	4	0–10	56–76
Alzheimer's disease and Downs syndrome	1	0	45
Frontotemporal dementia	1	0	90
Lewy body dementia	1	8	78
Dementia type unspecified	2	0, 17	92, 91

This procedure highlighted questions and statements that were unclear, ambiguous, or that consistently did not pick up any disability, as well as any areas of difficulty or management not currently included on the form. A literature search identified articles concerned with assessment and management of feeding or swallowing problems in this area. More studies were found regarding feeding than swallowing disorders, and studies varied considerably in the quality of their methodology and sample sizes. The literature was examined to see if any common areas of difficulty or management were omitted from the tool. The tool was then adapted accordingly, and the literature used to supplement the information found in this resource. This version was then sent to seven speech and language therapists experienced in working with people with dementia, with a questionnaire to identify any areas that were omitted or unclear. Using these comments the resource was then adapted into the final version printed here.

This resource is aimed at speech and language therapists who have little experience with dysphagia and dementia, and those with more experience who are interested in developing their knowledge with regard to the literature on eating and swallowing disorders in dementia. The assessment is designed to be used predominantly in long-term care environments such as nursing and residential homes, and in long-stay wards. It could also be used to assess people living in their own homes, looked after by relatives or carers. It will be relevant to other professionals working within the multi-disciplinary team who have an interest in dysphagia – eg, occupational therapists, dietitians and nurses.

The assessment has been produced in two formats:

1   *Format A*: a detailed format for less experienced therapists

2   *Format B*: a checklist format for more experienced therapists.

The history form should take on average 20 minutes to complete. Following on from this, the mealtime observation schedule is designed to be completed while observing the person at a mealtime. This should take no longer than 30 minutes, or as long as the mealtime. Once you have identified a problem area, possible management strategies have been provided (in detail in Chapter 4, and in checklist format in Chapter 6). The advice given is not designed to be prescriptive, because of the variability and complexity in the presentation of such problems in dementia. There are a range of possible strategies, and those professionals working closely with an affected individual will be able to use their knowledge of them and the eating environment to examine which may be successful. All staff working with this client group will recognise that management strategies are rarely total solutions, and are usually designed to minimise, rather than eliminate difficulties. As individuals deteriorate, the strategies used will need to change to meet those needs.

3

History-Taking –
Feeding and Swallowing Problems

The complete assessment profile is contained in Chapter 5, and the history form is the first part of it. The aim of this is to gather information regarding the development of the feeding and swallowing problem, and the factors that may have an impact upon it. This will help the team to identify the cause of the problem, and whether direct treatment is possible, or indirect management more appropriate. All too often in dementia, when there is a deterioration in the person's condition, it is assumed to be due to progression of the dementia. This may be right, but in some cases the change may be due to other factors, including co-occurring physical illness and mood disorder, which are open to intervention. Information may come from a variety of sources including staff, relatives and medical records. The following explains the history form.

Initially you are asked to note relevant professionals and carers:

Doctor. You will need to consult the doctor if you are concerned about the person's health or wellbeing; if you wish the person to be referred to other disciplines, or you need information regarding the person's past medical and psychiatric history.

Family/carers and professionals involved. A space has been included in which to note the family members involved, as well as any professionals, because these individuals may be a valuable source of information regarding current and past difficulties. In addition, as ethical issues are often involved, relatives may need to be consulted in the process of making decisions regarding feeding management.

You are then asked about the person's previous medical history:

Past medical and psychiatric history. You are asked to consider the person's previous medical and psychiatric history, to see if the difficulties are related to, or a reoccurrence of, a previous problem. It is worth noting the type of dementia they have, and considering if the difficulties presented are usually part of this condition (see Chapter 1). Note the presence of past chest infection, as you will need to consider if repeated chest infections are due to an underlying swallowing problem, causing chronic aspiration of food contents into the airway, and leading to infection (Logemann, 1983).

The questions listed below are to help you explore the possible reasons for the person's decline in eating and/or swallowing, and who you are likely to need to contact for further help.

1   *When did the eating/swallowing problem first start?*

    Consider if this is a new problem or long-standing. This is particularly relevant if the person has just been admitted to hospital, or a new care facility. Ask people who know the person best – maybe a relative. This will help establish if the problem is of a chronic or acute nature. Questions 2 and 3 also relate to this issue.

2   *Did it start gradually/suddenly?*

    If the problem started suddenly, you are advised to examine other events around this time to consider the cause. For example, a possible cause is a stroke, and this is obviously more likely in individuals suffering from a vascular dementia. Consider if there were other signs of stroke, such as facial or limb weakness, dysarthria or other communication problems. In some cases, problems of a more rapid onset may be due to co-occurring acute physical illness – for example, the person may have a chest or urinary infection; severe constipation can have significant effects on an individual's behaviour, including eating. Discuss the person's physical state with the nursing and medical staff involved.

    Gradual problems are more likely to be, but are not always due to the gradual progression of the dementia. In this case, consider if it fits with the person's general level of deterioration to date (see question 3) and is consistent with the type of dementia they have.

3   *Is the problem getting worse? If so, is it happening gradually or rapidly?*

    If the person is getting worse rapidly, you may need to seek further advice as a matter of urgency – for example, discussing with nursing staff, or contacting the doctor. Also note whether this is consistent with their general level of deterioration. For example, if a person has previously deteriorated in their dementia very slowly, and has then taken a rapid turn for the worse, you should consider if there are any other causes for this as well as their dementia – eg, physical illness or mood disorder.

4   Has the person experienced repeated chest infections in the past year?

Consider if repeated infections could be caused by underlying swallowing problems, and aspiration of food/fluid into the lungs. When you observe the person, pay particular attention to Sections 4 and 5 of the assessment, and explanatory notes, to highlight any possible swallowing problems. Find out about other factors that may affect their chest status, such as chronic chest complaints.

5   Has the person lost or gained weight?

Note weight now, and previous weights over the last 12 months, as well as reported usual weight from relatives.

It is common for people with dementia to lose weight as the dementia progresses, and it is often assumed that this always occurs in the later stages of the illness. However, Steele (1997) has highlighted the fact that those with mild to moderate impairment are at risk of poor intake, because they have to feed themselves and experience problems in this process. She therefore argues for more active intervention with this group. It is often hard to see if people are losing weight over time, and are at risk of nutritional deficiency. VOICES (1998) have therefore advised that residents should be weighed on admission to a nursing or residential home, and then on a monthly basis. They advise that those with a recent unintended weight loss or gain of 3 kg or more be referred for further advice from a health care professional, such as the doctor or dietitian. Plotting weight on a graph over time can be very helpful, as this may reveal a steady but dramatic loss. In some cases there is increase in weight due to overeating. This appears to be a stage that about a quarter of people with dementia go through (Trinkle *et al*, 1992). Bathgate *et al* (2001) found that overeating was part of a constellation of behavioural changes, particularly associated with frontotemporal dementia (Pick's disease). Other eating changes in this group included an altered preference for sweet foods; eating continually while food remains present; stealing from others' plates; seeking out food, and cramming food. In such cases, caregivers often need to restrict the type and amount of food taken.

6   Is the person diabetic? How is this controlled and monitored?

Ageing is associated with an increased prevalence of non-insulin dependent diabetes. Retrospective studies have indicated that good blood glucose control reduces the likelihood and severity of stroke, cardiovascular disease, visual impairment, nephropathy and infections, as well as cognitive dysfunction. Poor diabetic control can impact significantly on behaviour. Therefore, consider if the person's diabetes is stable over time and controlled appropriately. The person may not remember they are diabetic, so in care settings there should be a system of informing new or bank staff that a person is diabetic, and how this is managed. Any advice regarding food and drink for these individuals needs to take diabetic control into account.

7   ***Is the eating/swallowing problem variable from day to day, within the day or within the meal?***

You will need to consider why this might be. Is the person's general condition also variable? For example, some types of dementia are more fluctuating in their presentation – this is the case with dementia of the Lewy body type (McKeith, 1996). See Chapter 1 for further information on this condition; but the major feature of this illness is a fluctuating confusional state that can vary even from moment to moment.

Consider if the variability is related to environmental factors – eg, is the person worse when the dining-room is busier and more noisy? It could relate to the person's level of fatigue – eg, Suski (1989) has advised that optimum intake may be at the midday meal when individuals are at their best, and larger helpings should be given then. Some people may be tired by the end of the day, and take less of the evening meal. In the author's experience, this is highly variable, with some individuals being better at breakfast, and others less so. Some people may tire through the meal itself, with their performance deteriorating towards the end. You should also consider if the person eats more of one meal than another, and why this could be. For example, the dining area may be quieter and more relaxed at breakfast, or breakfast may be a softer and sweeter meal (such as cereal with sugar). You should also consider the effects of medication – eg, has the person been given medication which is likely to make them drowsy (see question 13). Some individuals given medication to help them sleep at night, for example, may still be under its effects in the morning, and as a result are less alert at breakfast. If you are concerned about this, discuss it with their doctor, nurse or psychiatrist to see if a reduction, or change, in the medication is appropriate. Charting the person's behaviour and oral intake may help to uncover reasons for any variability.

8   *Has there been a change in the person's level of consciousness and attention recently?*

See question 9 below.

9   *Has there been a change in the person's physical health recently?*

Physical illness, or metabolic disturbance, can affect the functioning of the nervous system, leading to an 'acute confusional state'. This can be caused by a variety of factors including infections – eg, of the chest and urinary tract; toxic states due to drug overdose, and liver and kidney dysfunction. The features of acute confusional state are outlined in Chapter 1. They include fluctuating level of arousal; disordered thought; erratic responses and evidence of physical disease on examination and laboratory investigations (Neary, 1999). This may have an obvious effect on an individual's feeding skills, and the risk of aspiration may be higher for these people, because of the fluctuations in arousal. Look for signs of co-occurring infection and, if necessary, request medical assessment and treatment.

10   *Has there been a change in the person's mood recently – eg, low in mood?*

Consider if a reduction in dietary intake may be due to a depressive illness, as reduced appetite is one of the biological features of depression (Martin, 1987). Look for other signs of depression (Goldberg *et al*, 1987):

Emotional changes:

◆ Loss of interest or pleasure in usual activities

◆ Feelings of sadness or hopelessness

◆ Crying spells

Cognitive changes:

◆ Feelings of self-dislike, guilt and worthlessness

◆ Difficulty thinking and making decisions

◆ Nihilistic ideas – eg, person feels they are already dead or have no feelings

◆ Thoughts of death or suicide attempts

Motivational changes:

◆ Low energy and apathy

◆ Fatigue

◆ Inability to concentrate

Neurovegetative symptoms:

◆ Disturbance in appetite

◆ Disturbance in sleep rhythm

◆ Diurnal variation of mood (in more severe cases), where mood is worst in the mornings.

In the elderly, depression may present particularly with perplexity; apparent lack of awareness and disregard of surroundings; slowing of speech, and movement and impaired concentration (Burns, 1995). At times this can be mistaken for dementia, and therefore is often termed 'pseudodementia'. People with dementia may also suffer from depression. This can be difficult to diagnose due to communication difficulties; however, observation of changes in behaviour is vital to this process. The reported prevalence of depressive symptoms in dementia varies considerably (0–87 per cent), but depressive disorders are less (10–24 per cent) (Allen & Burns, 1995).

If necessary, liaise with the doctor, or ask for the person to be referred to a psychiatrist. Cullen *et al* (1997) state that it is important to assess for depression in any person with dementia with a decreased food intake, because in their study, major depression was associated with decreased food consumption in some patients. Volicer *et al* (1994) demonstrate that treatment with antidepressants often improves food intake, even in individuals with severe dementia.

11 **Have there been changes in the person's behaviour of late – eg, disturbed or psychotic behaviour?**

Some individuals with psychiatric disturbance may experience an elevation of mood called 'mania'. Other symptoms of this include grandiose ideas, irritability, increased activity (involving motor behaviour, speech and thoughts), and disinhibition (Goldberg 1987). Individuals suffering from mania often do things quickly, including eating, and this can lead to coughing on food, due to cramming and poor chewing. Manic symptoms are reported less often than depression in dementia (5–17 per cent) (Allen & Burns, 1995), but may be a feature worth considering in long-term psychiatric patients who have co-occurring cognitive problems. Bazemore *et al* (1991), for example, highlighted 'fast eating syndrome' in a variety of psychiatric disorders.

Other people with dementia may develop abnormal beliefs about food – eg, that it is poison; that it does not belong to them; or that they do not deserve to eat it. Again, look at the person's history to see if they have suffered such difficulties before, and the features they displayed at this time. Liaise with the doctor, psychiatric nurse, or psychiatrist, as appropriate, because there may be treatment or management advice available for this.

12 **Does the person complain, or nonverbally indicate any pain or discomfort while eating?**

Pain is not commonly associated with neurological disorders of swallowing (Groher, 1997). If this occurs ask the doctor to examine the person. They may have a throat infection, such as tonsillitis, pharyngitis, or thrush, a mechanical obstruction or, more rarely, serious difficulties such as neoplasm. In clinical practice, the most commonly occurring difficulties are infections and thrush, individuals with the latter often complaining of severe pain, 'like swallowing razor blades', on swallowing. Some individuals may complain of food 'sticking', or discomfort when swallowing. This can be due to pharyngeal or oesophageal problems, and requires further assessment or investigation.

13 **(a) List the person's current medication**
    (b) Do any of these medications have any side effects that could affect movement, level of consciousness, concentration, appetite, saliva production, mood, or level of confusion?
    (c) Did the eating/swallowing problem occur after a change in medication?

List the medications and look them up in a relevant text, such as *The British National Formulary* (latest version), to see if side effects may be impacting on feeding or swallowing. A number of researchers have emphasised that swallowing problems can occur as a side effect of antipsychotic (also called neuroleptic) medication (eg, Sokoloff, 1997, and Bazemore, 1991). Such medications are described as having 'extra pyramidal' side effects – eg, Parkinsonism, akathisia or dystonia (explained below). Antipsychotics/neuroleptics are often used in dementia to control disturbed, disruptive or aggressive behaviour. Although this is not a common cause of swallowing problems, it is worth noting because the effect may be reversible (Stoschus, 1993). McKeith *et al* (1996) indicate that patients with Lewy body dementia may be particularly sensitive to this type of medication.

Parkinsonism mimics the effects of Parkinson's disease. There is rigidity in muscles, and in some cases tremor, leading to difficulties in initiation and control of movement. Severity ranges from barely perceptible absence of facial expression and stiffness of posture or gait, to complete immobility (Cookson *et al*, 1993). This can affect limbs, leading to problems with feeding, or can affect the muscles in the neck and throat, leading to difficulties with swallowing. Weeks may elapse from the start of the drug to the onset of symptoms, and so this may be a missed cause of any difficulties.

Dystonia is a distortion of posture, caused by involuntary contracture of one or more muscle groups – eg, there is spasm of the jaw, neck or spine. Acute dystonia comes on suddenly, occurring early in the course of drug treatment. There may be problems with swallowing, speaking or breathing as a result (Cookson *et al*, 1993).

Akathisia is a compulsive motor restlessness, especially of the legs (Cookson *et al*, 1993). This may lead to difficulties for the person in sitting for long enough to have a meal, or the associated mental agitation may cause them to be more confused.

Other side effects of antipsychotics may be a dry mouth, impaired concentration, increased confusion and sedation.

In some people, continuous treatment with antipsychotics can lead to 'Tardive Dyskinesia'. In this condition there are abnormal, involuntary movements of the extremities, trunk, neck and tongue, and these may not stop if medication is reduced or stopped. This condition is more common in long-term psychiatric patients. It may affect initiation or control of chewing or swallowing (Groher, 1997). Swallowing problems related to this condition have been termed 'dyskinetic dysphagia' (Bazemore *et al*, 1991).

There is also a condition known as 'Neuroleptic Malignant Syndrome', which is a very rare side effect of neuroleptics/antipsychotics. This consists of generalised muscular rigidity (which can make swallowing and breathing difficult), with pyrexia, autonomic instability, and lowered consciousness. Medication must be stopped immediately or the outcome may be fatal (Cookson *et al*, 1993).

There are a number of different antipsychotics, with differing properties. Some are more potent than others, and at an individual level people vary in their response to a given drug. The elderly and those with brain damage tend to be more susceptible to side effects (Cookson *et al*, 1993).

Commonly used antipsychotics in the elderly include:

◆ Haloperidol

◆ Promazine

◆ Sulperide

◆ Risperidone

◆ Olanzapine

◆ Chlorpromazine.

Some antidepressants may also have side effects that impact on eating. These include over-sedation, agitation, indigestion, nausea, dry mouth, constipation, dystonia and Parkinsonism. Each has its own constellation of possible side effects. Common antidepressants used in the elderly include:

◆ Amitriptyline

◆ Lofepramine

◆ Imipramine

◆ Clomipramine

◆ Dothiepin

◆ Trazodone

◆ Fluoxetine

◆ Paroxetine

◆ Citalopram

◆ Sertraline.

If you are concerned about possible side effects, talk to the person's nurse, doctor, or pharmacist.

4

Assessment and Management of Feeding and Swallowing

The complete assessment profile is printed in two versions in Chapter 5. The sections and questions in this chapter refer to those used in the 'mealtime observation schedule', which is the second part of the assessment. This chapter outlines the difficulties often presented at mealtimes by individuals with dementia. Research evidence, where available, is used to explain such problems and ways to manage them. Case studies from the author's clinical experience are used to illustrate the points made. Relevant management strategies are summarised in checklist form in Chapter 6, for greater ease of use.

This chapter is divided into assessment and management of the following:

1   Sensory impairment and dentition

2   Mental state and behaviour

3   Feeding situation and skills

4   Issues related to food/drink and swallowing

5   Severe swallowing problems.

There is overlap between these sections, and in some respects divisions are fairly arbitrary. However, attempts have been made to cross reference areas where relevant.

1 Assessment and management issues related to sensory impairment and dentition

Sensory impairment and dentition may seem too obvious to mention. However, in the author's experience, they may be overlooked, and because there are at least partial solutions to these problems they are included here. Difficulties in these areas can affect self-feeding skills, in the case of vision; and the person's response while being fed, in the case of hearing. Given the level of visual and auditory impairment in the elderly (Grimes, 1995), it is worth checking that any sensory deficits are corrected if possible. Difficulties with dentition can have significant effects on eating, and again may go unrecognised. Each question is considered in turn.

1(a) Does the person have visual difficulties?

For example, do they need glasses or have problems with the ones they have, or have cataract, hemianopia or visual neglect?

If the person has glasses, find out when they should be wearing them. Are they just for reading, or should they have them on all the time, including at meals? When people become confused, they often mix up old and new pairs of glasses, and those for reading and distance, and it can be a problem finding the correct pair. Relatives may be able to help. Ensure that glasses are clean and fit properly. The person may not be aware that their glasses do not fit and constantly slide down their nose, so that they are looking through the frame or over the top. This is more common in those who have a stooped posture. Ensure all who are involved know that the person should wear their glasses.

There are other visual problems that may interfere with eating, including: cataract, hemianopia (only seeing one side of the visual field) and visual neglect (neglecting one side of the body and the environment). The latter two features may occur in the context of stroke. For these people, caregivers may need to draw their attention to items on the table, or put utensils directly into their hands. Such individuals may only 'see' one side of their plate, and only eat the food there. They need their plate turned for them during the meal.

For individuals who are being fed, consider the feeder's position. If the person neglects one side, the feeder should not sit there to feed, but place themself just off-centre on their 'good' side. Ensure that the lighting is good, and that the feeder sits facing the light or window so that their face is not in shadow.

The case study of 'Susan' on page 28 highlights how vision can affect a variety of skills, including feeding.

Susan

Susan had chronic mental health problems and had lived in different institutions for much of her adult life. Now elderly, she was developing memory problems, and had become increasingly withdrawn and less communicative, spending much of the time with her eyes closed and her arms tightly folded. She needed help with all activities of daily living, and could no longer feed herself. She had cataracts in both eyes, and her sister felt that an operation to remove these would be of great benefit.

Following the surgery it turned out that Susan's sister had been correct. Within two weeks of the operation, Susan was much brighter in her mood and was taking in her surroundings. She was not only responding to communication, but was also initiating it. Four weeks later she was able to feed herself again. Susan continued to suffer from memory problems, and sometimes confusion, but the cataract surgery radically changed her quality of life and ability to engage in skills of everyday living.

Such a success may be rare, but it is worth noting that we often attribute deterioration to progression of dementia, and therefore feel that it is not remediable. Yet in some cases this deterioration may be due to other factors that are open to change and treatment.

If there are significant visual problems, utensils and cups should be placed directly into the person's hands at each stage of the meal. They should be told about the food or drink. Consider referring them to an occupational therapist, with a view to obtaining aids for the visually impaired, if their difficulties impact significantly on eating.

If you suspect that a person's vision needs to be assessed, or that a stronger or different prescription is necessary, refer them to an optician. If you are worried that they may not be able to cooperate with the procedure, discuss this with the optician, do not just give up. If you are concerned about cataracts, discuss this with their doctor or optician.

1(b) Does the person need a hearing aid, or is the one they have not working?

If the person has a hearing aid, ensure that they are wearing it and that it is turned on. The ear mould should be cleaned regularly of wax, by wiping it each night when it is removed or, if it has become clogged, by unscrewing the mould from the aid and soaking it in warm, lightly soaped water. Batteries should be checked regularly. The aid should be on the correct setting, usually mid volume. If it is whistling in the person's ear, turn down the volume. If you suspect the aid is not working, or the mould is faulty, contact your local Audiology department. Ensure that everyone involved is aware that the person should wear their aid, which ear it goes in, and how it works. If possible, discretely label the aid with an 'L' or 'R' on the inner side.

If you suspect the person has a hearing loss, but does not have an aid, discuss this with their nurse or doctor. It may be worth checking first to see if the person has impacted wax in their ears, and treating for this. If necessary, they should be referred to the local Ear, Nose and Throat, or Audiology department for a hearing test. There should be a care plan detailing management of the person's hearing loss and communication, and the speech and language therapist can give advice for this.

1(c) Does the person have problems with dentition – eg, need dentures or have problems with their dentures; have infected teeth, poor oral hygiene, or a sore mouth?

It is extremely important to consider dentition. People who do not have their own teeth are more likely to have poor nutritional status (Walls *et al*, 1997). Following weight loss, dentures may become ill-fitting and actually interfere with eating (eg, Carlsson, 1984; Smith, 1979). You should consider the use of denture fixative, or it may be necessary to consult with a dentist so that loose dentures can be adjusted or replaced. Many dentists will visit people's homes, or care homes. The British Relatives Association publication *Dental Care for Older People in Homes* (1995) provides information on dental care in Britain.

You should consider if the texture of the food is appropriate. If a person is unable or unwilling to wear dentures, they may not be able to chew all solid food – for example, stringy meat and fibrous vegetables – and so you may have to make some changes in their diet to take account of this. Equally, the fact that someone has no teeth or dentures, does not mean they need a liquidised diet. A great deal of chewing can be achieved by the gums and the tongue, mashing food against the hard palate.

Some people may retain a few of their own teeth. However, as the dementia has progressed, they may not have paid attention to their oral hygiene. Teeth may have become infected or loose. This can cause discomfort, and impair the taste of food. Those with advanced dementia may not be able to indicate this pain to others, and it may manifest itself in more generalised ways, affecting mood and behaviour. Ensure that staff and carers are aware that regular mouth care should be carried out, particularly for those who have oral residue or pocketing of food in their cheeks. If you are concerned, you should refer the person to the dentist. For those with behavioural problems, think of ways to help them engage in the dental assessment, perhaps by considering the location and time of the appointment, or by asking a relative to be present to reduce anxiety. In some cases, short-acting medication may be required to calm the person. Discuss such cases with the person's nurse or doctor.

2 Assessment and management issues related to mental state and behaviour

This section examines the person's mental state, and behavioural aspects that may affect feeding and swallowing.

2(a) Does the person have a reduced level of consciousness – are they drowsy?

An initial consideration should be to ascertain whether the person is alert enough to eat and drink. Those who are drowsy are likely to have difficulty eating and drinking adequate amounts. They may be at risk of aspiration due to a poor swallow, reduced cough reflex, or falling asleep with food in the oral cavity that could then be breathed in. It is worth considering if the person is physically ill in any way – eg, chest and urinary infections are common problems in the elderly – or has suffered a stroke. If they have not been assessed already, discuss this with their nurse, or consult the doctor. If they are believed to be in the terminal stages of dementia, refer to Parts 4 and 5 of this chapter for further information.

Also consider if the drowsiness could be a side effect of any medication. In this case, there may be a pattern to the problem. Chapter 3, question 13 of the history section, discussed side effects of medication. Fatigue may also be a factor: some people may tire significantly through the day, and eat less as the day goes on. Consider if they could be given extra helpings when they are alert, or if their food needs to be fortified so they receive extra nutrition. Is there flexibility within the feeding routine to provide something to eat outside set mealtimes? If the person is taking only fluids, a supplement drink should be considered, rather that just tea (Volicer, 1998). Consult their doctor or the dietitian with regard to this.

The person should be fed in as upright a posture as possible, and only when they are alert enough to chew and swallow safely. Particular attention should be paid to ensure that their mouth is clear of food at the end of a meal, and regular mouth care is given.

2(b) Is it difficult to get the person to sit for any length of time at the table?

Wandering is a common problem in dementia. Often the drive to wander is so great that it overrides the concentration needed to eat. In addition, individuals with dementia may have marked communication problems affecting expressive skills and understanding (Hart, 1990). They may not understand when told it is a mealtime, and may need extra nonverbal prompts, or indeed be shown the food to understand that they need to sit down. The person may keep getting up from the table if the food has yet to arrive. Therefore, it may be better to let them wander, and then bring them to the table when the meal is ready, giving them the appropriate verbal and nonverbal prompts at this time. Be wary of assuming that the person does not like the food, or has finished. They may need encouragement to come back to the table – eg, 'John... you've got some pudding here... sit here.' You are likely to need to use additional verbal and nonverbal prompts, and even in some instances to sit down on a chair nearby while gesturing to the chair next to you, to show the person what you mean. It may be necessary to give extra helpings of food when they are more settled.

Kline and Sexton (1996) observed 37 individuals who displayed agitation. They found that this often had an adverse effect on mealtimes. They were concerned to note that those who showed the greatest frequency of agitated behaviour during meals were often given only minimal amounts of verbal encouragement or touch, even when meals were poorly eaten.

Such people may be able to feed themselves, but are in need of cues to encourage them to eat adequately. Kline and Sexton advocate that nursing homes pay special attention to recognising the difficulties of these individuals. VOICES (1998) suggest that for those who cannot sit for long to eat, finger foods that can be eaten on the move should be provided.

It is worth considering the cause of any agitation: is it due solely to the dementia? In some instances it may be due to the side effects of medication, or co-occurring acute physical illness. It will be worth finding out about the onset and evolution of any behavioural disturbance, and discussing with other team members to ascertain if further advice or assessment is required.

2(c) Does the person forget what they are doing, or become distracted from the task?

This question is related to 2(b), so also refer to the information there. People with dementia may be easily distracted, or have problems with 'immediate memory', which leads to difficulty in keeping track of the task in hand (Snowden, 1999). The latter is particularly associated with Alzheimer's disease. Typically, at mealtimes a person may start to eat, but then become distracted or stop eating because they have lost track of, or forgotten, what they were doing. They may start fiddling with something at the table, or just get up and wander away. Gentle prompts to continue are often effective – eg, either verbal prompts, or gently sitting the person back down and putting the utensil back in their hand.

It is worth considering the level of distractions in the dining area. Is the person being distracted by other residents; by people walking through, or by the general noise level? Are there ways to reduce these distractions? Is there part of the dining area that has fewer distractions, away from the door or serving hatch perhaps? Consider the noise level: is there loud music playing; a television on, or plates banging? Could a calmer atmosphere be conveyed? Ragneskog *et al* (1996) videotaped five people with dementia in a nursing home at mealtimes, and found that playing calming music affected behaviour. For example, four out of five people spent more time at the table, and appeared calmer. They postulated that soothing music reduced restlessness and anxiety. Denney (1997) showed a reduction in agitated behaviours at mealtimes when quiet music was played, in a sample of nine people with dementia. When this music was withdrawn, behaviours rebounded, only to decline again with reintroduction of the music. Therefore, reducing agitation at mealtimes may have a positive effect on oral intake. It is important that the music played reflects the needs and preferences of residents, and not of staff.

2(d) Is the person very passive? Do they need prompts to start eating?

Some people may be very passive and require external prompts to start eating. As suggested above, such prompts may be verbal or physical. For example, you could put the utensil in their hand and guide them to start, or even give them the first mouthful. There is some evidence that people with dementia will look to those around them for cues (Priefer, 1997). Some people may therefore be helped by sitting with others who are more able, and who they can copy. If their self-feeding is erratic, sometimes they may need to be fed at least part of their meal. Some people may need prompting to move from one course to the next (Osborne & Marshall, 1993).

It is important to consider why a person is so passive. It could be due to the dementia, but think too if it could be due to depression (see Chapter 3, question 10 for further information).

For some people with dementia, signs of hunger or thirst may not be felt in the normal way, or expressed. For these people there is no build-up to eating: food suddenly arrives. Mealtime cues can be increased by talking about food or, in some instances, by getting the people to help sort out or lay the table. This can increase the pleasure experienced at mealtimes, and may be a good source of social contact and stimulation.

2(e) Does the person refuse food or drink? Do they verbally refuse; push the food or feeder away; keep their mouth shut; turn their head away; spit food out; hit out, etc?

For those who need to be fed, there may be the problem of food refusals, or spitting out food, etc (Athlin & Norberg, 1987a). Those feeding themselves may verbally refuse food and push it away. However, Osborn and Marshall (1993) found that some self-feeding individuals may verbally say 'no', but with verbal and physical encouragement, may behaviourally say 'yes'. It is important to remember that food refusals are unlikely to be the person being 'difficult': it may not necessarily be an active decision on their part to refuse food; there are likely to be reasons for this, related either to their dementia, or to other co-occurring conditions. For example, oral apraxia may mean that the person is unable to volitionally open their mouth to a spoon or cup; or once food is introduced, they may be unable to move it around, or to initiate a swallow (Blandford *et al*, 1998). This can occur in the absence of significant oral weakness. Others will be better once they have tasted the meal: they may not understand that someone was trying to feed them. Try putting a small amount of food on their lips, or gently resting the spoon there, giving verbal prompts and encouragement to open their mouth. Assess if the person is better at opening their mouth to a spoon or a cup, and start with the easiest, until they have got into the task. One carer the author worked with found that his wife, who had oral apraxia, had particular problems opening her mouth at the start of a meal. He found that she was better at drinking than eating, so used a successful strategy of starting the meal with a few mouthfuls of fluid to get her into the task before moving on to diet. Others may have the reverse pattern. The person may be better if they can be involved in the feeding process, either by self-feeding if possible, or by holding the cup or spoon while the caregiver guides it to their mouth. Experiment with different tastes and temperatures to see if this elicits a better swallow. Rather than direct prompts, indirect cues such as talking about the food may help – 'that tastes nice', etc.

Basavaraju (1981) points out that in the later stages of dementia, primitive reflexes may emerge that interfere with eating. For example, the person may bite on the spoon as the bite reflex has been evoked, and this may be misinterpreted as a refusal to eat.

In one of her case studies, Kayser-Jones (1996) raises the possibility that sometimes turning the head away can be a strategy that individuals with swallowing difficulty may use as a protective measure, to give them time to swallow before taking another mouthful. This is often observed by speech and language therapists. Such behaviour may not be a conscious strategy, just an indication that the person is not ready to continue eating. They may therefore need a slower feeding rate.

Infected and painful teeth can influence eating and cooperation at mealtimes (see Section 1(c) for further information).

You may find that some members of staff are more successful than others at getting the person to eat. It is therefore worth observing or discussing feeding technique in order to consider the reasons for this. In some cases it may be helpful to chart the refusals, to see if any patterns emerge. It is important to record when and where the meal was taken; what the meal was; how much was eaten, and the person's behaviour and any verbalisations at refusal. It is also worth noting any effects of the environment at such times. Using this approach, you can see if there are any patterns to the food refusal, such as the time of day, food types or tastes.

Many people with dementia experience a change in their food preferences, and many develop a particular liking for sweet food (Mungas *et al*, 1990) and refuse food of a savoury nature. Some dislike bitty foods – eg, hard minced meat – and spend the meal removing each bit from their mouth or spitting it out, often giving up before the food is eaten. A softer and smoother texture may be appropriate.

The thoughts and beliefs of a person with dementia may be confused because they do not recognise where they are now, or the associated routine, and are therefore fearful and uncertain. Some people may behave as though they are reliving events from the past. Strategies to help them may concentrate not necessarily on the food, but on addressing these beliefs. The case study of Mrs Griffiths illustrates this.

Mrs Griffiths

Mrs Griffiths, who suffered from Alzheimer's disease, came into hospital from a residential home, due to weight loss and refusal to eat. Initial food charts did not reveal any pattern to this problem, apart from a mild suggestion that she preferred sweet things, and therefore yielded no solutions. However, the charts were then expanded to include Mrs Griffiths' behaviour and verbalisations at mealtimes. Analysis of these revealed that Mrs Griffiths repeatedly stated that she did not want anything to eat, because she could not afford it, as she had no money in her purse. She tried to give her food away to staff sitting with her, often saying 'Why aren't you having any, love?'. She would often get up during a meal to go to the toilet, and then refuse to sit back at the table. Discussion with Mrs Griffiths' daughter revealed that since her dementia Mrs Griffiths had become focused on the cost of things, and was anxious if she could not remember if she had paid for something.

To manage such difficulties, Mrs Griffiths was prompted to use the toilet before each mealtime. She was guided to sit at the table, and told that this meal was for her, and that she had already paid for it (this information was repeated at intervals during the meal). A member of staff sat with her, and had their own drink and small snack. Reassurance was given when she became anxious, and if she tried to give her food to staff, they declined, saying they had their own. As Mrs Griffiths also had some spatial problems and distractibility leading to difficulty feeding, she was given only one course at a time with a fork, and all other distractions were removed. If she really did not want to eat, a supplement milk shake drink was given along with snacks between meals. Mrs Griffiths significantly increased the amount of food she was taking and stopped losing weight. These strategies were relayed to the residential home where she returned.

In their survey *Food for Thought*, the Alzheimer's Society (2000) found that a number of carers reported that the colour of food had become more important to people with dementia – with bright red or orange foods being particularly appealing. They speculated that this may be due to vision being affected in dementia. The author has worked with a woman with Alzheimer's disease who would eat only white food, presenting quite a problem at mealtimes.

There may be other reasons why individuals do not eat, related either to depression, or to holding abnormal beliefs about the food. Volicer (1994) found that treatment with antidepressant medication was effective not only in improving the mood of demented patients, but also in improving their food intake. Depression can be difficult to diagnose in people with advanced dementia, but it is treatable, so contact the person's doctor if you suspect this is the case (see Chapter 3, question 10 for further information on depression). Some individuals may hold abnormal beliefs about food – eg, that it is poison, or that it has been tampered with in some way. Such suspicious or delusional ideas are not uncommon in dementia. Find out if the person has had such ideas in the past, and how they were treated – for example, by asking their doctor, psychiatric nurse or psychiatrist. Consider ways of combating these beliefs. One woman with dementia would eat only if the food was opened and prepared in front of her. Others may respond to verbal reassurance and explanation.

2(f) Is the speed of eating or drinking inappropriate?

Too fast

Ask staff if this is a typical pattern at mealtimes and not just because of hunger. Bazemore *et al* (1991) discuss 'fast eating syndrome' in respect of patients with psychiatric problems, and this behaviour can occur in dementia. Bathgate *et al* (2001) found that eating fast and cramming food was often a feature of frontotemporal dementia. In this condition, individuals may lack the judgement to know how much to put in their mouths at once. They may put in unmanageable amounts and this, coupled with poor chewing, can lead to choking. Such people will need their food cut up into small pieces. Do this before you give them their meal, not in front of them, to preserve dignity. They should be supervised when eating, so they cannot cram food. Verbal prompts to slow down may be effective, but it is often necessary for staff to gently put their hand on the person's hand, to stop them taking more before they are ready. Try serving each course in a number of smaller portions, with a short gap between each, to give time for chewing and swallowing any crammed food. A softer and more moist diet may be necessary, if their chewing is poor, to reduce choking on food. For some, the environment and level of distractions – for example, the noise level – may exacerbate the situation. If so, the environment should be altered accordingly, perhaps by reducing background noise or by playing gentle music.

Mr Hobbs' case, illustrates management of 'fast eating syndrome' in an individual with both vascular dementia and mania (see Chapter 3, question 11 for further information on the latter).

Mr Hobbs

Mr Hobbs had a vascular dementia and a history of persistent mania. When he was suffering a manic episode, he would become very agitated, and at such times could not sit to eat. Even during stable periods when he could sit down, he would eat very quickly, putting large amounts of food in his mouth – eg, cramming in a whole potato, and then trying to eat another. His chewing was poor, and this led to coughing and choking.

Staff managed this problem by avoiding hard or chewy foods; by cutting his food into small pieces, and by ensuring there was more moisture in his food, in the form of gravy or sauce. Mr Hobbs was verbally prompted to slow down by a member of staff who sat with him and, if necessary, the member of staff would gently stop him taking another mouthful and encourage him to chew and swallow what was already in his mouth.

Too slow

Some people with dementia eat very slowly. In this case you need to see if there are ways that the meal can be kept hot and appetising, perhaps by serving courses separately, or in smaller helpings. You may wish to use a heat retaining plate (warmed not hot), which can be obtained through an occupational therapist, who may also be helpful if you are concerned that feeding difficulties are causing the person to eat slowly. If they also take only small amounts of diet, consider whether this will maintain their nutritional status. Ensure that food is high in calories, and give snacks between meals. It may be necessary to feed the person the second half of their meal, if this a serious problem. Records should be kept regarding the amount the person eats and their weight. If you are concerned about their intake, ask their doctor to refer them to the dietitian.

Some individuals suffering from depression become withdrawn and slowed in all their activities of daily living, including eating (see Chapter 3, question 10). Consult their doctor if you are concerned they may be depressed.

2(g) Does the person eat non-food items?

There have been a number of reports of people with dementia eating inappropriate substances, including uncooked foods and disgusting or dangerous non-food items such as tissues and faeces. Morris (1989) describes this behaviour and discusses possible causes for it. With such people, all members of staff and carers should be alerted so that they can pay particular attention to this. The environment should be modified as much as possible, to remove any harmful substances such as cleaning fluids that may be drunk. Health and safety regulations control possible harmful substances in hospitals and nursing homes, and strict adherence to these will reduce the risks. At mealtimes, all non-food items may need to be removed – eg, tissues from the person's hands – to stop these being consumed with the food. There are a number of anecdotal reports that people with dementia may not have the usual response to painful or unpleasant stimuli. Therefore they may not spit out material that is burning or hurting the mouth.

3 Assessment and management issues related to feeding situation and skills

The general environment

This section relates to the person's skills in feeding, and if they cannot do this independently, how they are fed by staff, as well as wider issues relating to the mealtime environment.

Section 2 looked particularly at the effects of the environment on mood and behaviour, so there is some overlap here. A number of studies have focused on improving the eating environment. Better seating arrangements can enhance socialisation at mealtimes – for example, seating people at small tables rather than side by side (Davies & Snaith, 1980) – and can provide an environment where the more able residents can help the less able, by opening cartons, pouring, etc. Melin and Gotestam (1981) showed that organising coffee breaks and mealtimes around small tables, with greater choice and opportunity for self-service, aided both communication and eating behaviour. As stated in Chapter 3, Ragneskog *et al* (1996) found that playing appropriate music at mealtimes improved behaviour and oral intake. They postulated that soothing music reduced restlessness and anxiety. Denney (1997) also showed a reduction in agitated behaviours at mealtimes when quiet music was played. Eaton *et al* (1986) studied 21 individuals with dementia and 21 controls, and found that appropriate use of touch by staff at mealtimes, together with verbal encouragement, significantly improved on nutritional intake. Basic problems, such as cups that are out of reach or empty, have been identified in a hospital environment (Spencer *et al*, 2000).

Watson (1993) reviewed a range of issues in the feeding situation, including the difficulty of measuring the success of nursing interventions. He advised that single-case studies should be used for investigating feeding difficulty. To do this it is necessary to have a good description, not only of the difficulties a person experiences, but also of their environment, and how they are currently managed by staff in this setting. The following procedure is therefore suggested.

First, examine the general environment at mealtimes. Is the atmosphere calm and relaxed, or is it noisy and rushed? Are people allowed to take their time over eating, or do they have to finish within a specified time? Are there adjustments that could be made to make the mealtime more pleasurable? A typical example is in hospital wards, where patients are served food on a tray. For those with dementia this can be a confusing experience. The person may be faced with two courses, a roll wrapped in cling film, orange juice in a plastic pot that looks like a yoghurt, a cup of tea, a knife, fork and spoon, and a menu. It is little wonder that they do not know where to start, and often fiddle with food or attempt to 'eat' orange juice with a spoon. To keep the person focused, it is best to give them one course at a time, with just the relevant cutlery provided, and to reduce all other distractions. They should be asked if they want salt and pepper or sauce, and helped with this if necessary. Food should be removed from wrappers and drinks served in glasses. If the person cannot read the menu, they should be told what has been ordered. If they find the menu distracting, it should be removed. For many with dementia, just leaving a meal is unlikely to be successful. Prompting and encouragement are required.

Plain, light coloured tablecloths have been suggested by many to be better than brightly patterned ones, as cutlery can be seen more easily against a plain background by those with visual or spatial impairment. Consider the crockery and cutlery available. Elderly people often find small handles on cups and cutlery hard to hold. This is particularly true for those with arthritis or any limb weakness. Contrasting, plain, non-slip mats are useful to keep the plate in place.

Use the following prompts to help structure your observation of the mealtime situation.

3(a) Is the level of mealtime supervision inadequate?

It is important to consider if there is sufficient supervision at mealtimes, given the level of difficulty that the person may experience. Although many will not need feeding, they are certain to need prompts to help organise themselves with utensils, and to keep their attention on the task in hand. Steele (1997), in a large nursing home study, found that oral intake was actually poorer in those with mild to moderate impairment than those with more advanced dementia (as the latter group was fed). She argues that there is a need for more active intervention with this milder group.

Osborne and Marshall (1993) observed 23 residents in a nursing home at mealtimes, and found that some were are able to partially feed themselves. Rather than resort totally to spoon-feeding, they advocated the use of graded assistance. They developed a system of prompts ranging from unassisted, through verbal, to nonverbal prompts, and finally physical guidance, before full assistance in feeding is required. They also found that there are often differences in ability with self-feeding diet versus fluids. Individuals may, for example, be able to drink from a cup themselves, but be unable to feed themselves solids with or without utensils. People with dementia may also require prompting to move from one course to the next. Coyne and Hoskins (1997) examined the effects of verbal prompting and positive reinforcement on the level of eating independence of 24 elderly individuals with dementia, in a randomised control study. They found significant differences in eating performance when such prompts were given, and that this improvement was retained at a follow-up seven days later. They argue that a diagnosis of dementia should not preclude the possibility that eating skills may be reacquired.

A number of authors have therefore highlighted an 'all or nothing' approach to feeding. Individuals are perceived as either needing to be fed by a member of staff, or as independent in eating, whereas in reality there is a range of difficulties between these two poles (Kayser-Jones & Schell, 1997). By providing verbal and physical assistance, a great deal of difference can be made to the pleasure experienced at mealtimes, and also to the amount of diet taken. Consider if this type of help is available and is recognised as a need. It may take some reorganisation to achieve the required level of supervision, and low staffing levels are often a reason why this cannot be achieved. Osborn and Marshall (1993) suggest one way round this would be to assign a single staff member to assist a group of partially dependent residents in need of verbal, and occasional physical, help. Seating of residents may also be relevant, as less dependent individuals may naturally help the less able by handing them utensils and cups, and opening tops, etc.

Burton-Jones (1998) writes on behalf of the British Residents Association, arguing that relatives can provide a valuable source of information regarding a person's eating habits and preferences. The Association encourages relatives to be consulted about such issues and, where appropriate, to be invited to play an active part in feeding the person when they visit. This can be therapeutic for both parties involved, particularly when the person is advanced in their dementia and has little communication. The speech and language therapist may need to give both advice and training to relatives. Mr Edwards' case study illustrates the importance of adequate supervision.

Mr Edwards

Mr Edwards was in his fifties and suffered from Alzheimer's disease. Initially he had presented not with memory problems, but with spatial difficulties, and as his illness progressed this problem increasingly interfered with his activities of daily living. His spatial problems became so severe that he almost appeared blind. At mealtimes he could not use a knife and fork together, and found it difficult to locate the utensils, cups or food in front of him. He often ate from only one side of his plate. He knocked things over and was messy when eating. In contrast to this, his memory and insight into his condition were much less impaired. For example, he could tell you he had Alzheimer's, and how it affected him. His case illustrates that difficulties with feeding do not occur just in significantly confused individuals.

To reduce the difficulties presented, Mr Edwards was given only a fork or spoon, and all his food was cut up for him. Bitty food, or foods that would roll off a fork or spoon (eg, peas) were avoided. A plate guard was used to ensure food did not spill on to the table. Someone sat with him at mealtimes to ensure that any utensil, cup, or piece of food was placed directly into his hand, so he did not have to locate them himself. During the meal, food was gathered from around the plate to make sure he could find it. When he ate from one side of his plate, this was turned around for him. At all times he was given prompts, in a gentle but matter of fact manner, to preserve his dignity. This help ensured Mr Edwards was able to eat his meal more successfully, and reduced the distress and embarrassment he felt.

3(b) Is there a problem with the person's position when eating? For example, are they not fully upright, or is the table or chair not the correct height?

It is extremely important that any resident who is being fed is as upright in posture as possible (Kolodny & Malek, 1991). Steele *et al* (1997) found that 35 per cent of their nursing home sample had positioning problems. If such residents are not upright when eating and drinking, any swallowing problems are likely to be worse – for example, increasing coughing on food or fluid – and risk aspiration into the airway. The head and trunk should be in an upright position, and so for those with poor head or trunk control, a dining chair or wheelchair with no supports is not appropriate. It may therefore be better for the person to be fed in an upright lounge chair, with their head and trunk supported with pillows. Try to avoid feeding people in bed or on a bean bag, as it is often hard to maintain an upright posture. Think if there is appropriate seating that could be used instead, or if they need to be fed in such a way, methods should be explored to provide support, using extra pillows, etc. It is particularly in the later stages of dementia that problems maintaining posture are likely to occur. Some people may have stiffness and contracture of the limbs, and may require advice from the physiotherapist on seating and postural support. Occasionally individuals may have a habitual head posture with their chin resting on their chest, which makes feeding very difficult. Ask the physiotherapist for advice as to how to support the head in a more upright position.

The case of Miss Miles highlights the issue of adequate seating, particularly for people with more advanced dementia.

Miss Miles

Miss Miles suffered from Alzheimer's disease and was in the later stages of the illness. She could no longer weight bear, slid down most chairs and suffered from contractures of her limbs. However, her swallowing was much worse when she was not upright, and at these times she often coughed on her food. The physiotherapist assessed her and ordered an appropriate chair to support her. This made mealtimes much better for both Miss Miles and the staff feeding her, as she was able to maintain a more upright posture in her chair and coughed far less. In addition, she could also see what was going on around her throughout the day, and this increased her stimulation from the environment.

For those who are self-feeding, you need to consider if the chair and table are at the right height. This is often a problem if people are sitting in wheelchairs and cannot get close enough to the table. They should be mobilised into more appropriate seating, the wheelchair adjusted, or a fixed tray attached to their chair. People who are too far away from the table are likely to be messy, and this exacerbates feeding difficulties.

3(c) Does the person have difficulty self-feeding – for example, using or locating utensils or crockery on the table?

People with dementia gradually lose the ability to feed themselves as their illness progresses. Volicer *et al* (1987) found that in Alzheimer's disease, 50 per cent of people had lost the ability to feed themselves eight years after diagnosis. Typically, people start with difficulty using a knife and fork together, so they move on to using just a fork or spoon until eventually this becomes problematic. At the same time they may also be messy with their eating, and not be aware of this. It can be distressing for relatives, as there are certain social expectations around eating, and to see their loved one violate these and become almost childlike in their eating habits, is often a shock.

Two areas of cognitive difficulty that are particularly relevant to the skill of using cutlery are apraxia and spatial dysfunction. Apraxia refers to difficulty in carrying out purposeful sequences of movement voluntarily, despite normal primary motor skills (Hart, 1990). Various types of apraxia are reported in the literature. LeClerc *et al* (1998) describe how 'ideational apraxia' may affect self-feeding in Alzheimer's disease. They define ideational apraxia as loss of ability to conceptualise, plan and execute a complex sequence of motor actions involving the use of tools or objects, in spite of adequate muscle power, sensation and coordination. With respect to eating, this impairs a person's ability to initiate and sequence the actions required at mealtimes to use a knife, fork and spoon. In dementia, the person experiences increasing difficulty with this sequence of actions, and eating can become very frustrating for them.

Spatial function refers to the ability to locate things in space and orientate them correctly (Snowden, 1999). People with Alzheimer's disease in particular may have spatial problems.

For example, they may show difficulty in locating their knife/fork or cup, despite it being right in front of them, and may hold utensils the wrong way round, or put cups on to their food or the edge of the table. Mr Edwards in 3(a) (page 42) is an example of someone with spatial difficulties.

People with such problems will need to move from using a knife and fork to using only a fork or spoon with each meal. Food should be cut up for them, before giving them their meal, to maintain dignity. They should also be given one course at a time, and only the utensil they currently need, put directly into their hand. They should be asked if they want salt and pepper, sauce, etc and helped with this. A plate guard may be useful to stop food falling off the edge of the plate, or use a large bowl instead. Ensure a non-slip mat is placed under their plate, or a piece of thin, non-slip rubber. Consider if those with poor grip need cutlery or crockery with larger handles. Refer to the occupational therapist if you feel the person needs an assessment of their feeding skills and would benefit from feeding aids such as adapted cutlery.

Such people are likely to be able to feed themselves if they are given this help, together with adequate supervision, throughout the meal. For example, they may need help locating a glass from which to drink, or getting a utensil correctly orientated. They may lose track of what they are doing and require prompting to pick up cutlery again and continue. Some may need help to start the task – for example, help in holding the utensil and then guiding their hand to the food and their mouth, until they have got into the task. Prompts may be both verbal and physical. By breaking down the task like this, and providing the necessary help, staff can enable the person to maintain and enhance their eating skills (LeClerc, 1998).

Ford (1996) has described a 'Dementia Diet', outlining foods that can be eaten using only the hands, thus eliminating difficulties with cutlery. It may be well worth considering such 'finger foods' if the person is able to chew and swallow such textures. VOICES (1998) have adapted these into a list as shown in Table 4.1 (page 46).

TABLE 4.1 **DEMENTIA DIET: FINGER FOODS**

Breads and cereals	Vegetables
buttered toast/crumpet	carrot sticks or coins, cooked
rolls/muffins with butter	broccoli spears, cooked
sandwiches (not overfilled)	Brussels sprouts, cooked
crackers with butter	cauliflower pieces
biscuits with butter	green beans, cooked
buttered buns	chips
French toast	potato waffles
fruit loaf	new potatoes
fruit cake	sweet potato coins
teabread	fried battered onion rings
gingerbread	fried plantain
waffles	fried, crumbed whole mushrooms
dropscones	sliced cucumber
cereal bars	quartered tomato
chapattis/nan bread	celery sticks
small pittas	
won-tons	
prawn crackers	

Meat, fish, cheese and other protein alternatives	Fruit
sliced meat cut up into pieces	banana
chicken fingers from moist breast	melon
sausage and frankfurters	sliced apple or pear
hamburgers	strawberries
meatballs	grapes
meatloaf	pear halves
pizza	mandarin orange segments
slices of pork pie	
mini samosas	
mini spring rolls	**Snacks**
quiche	dried apricots and prunes (remove stones)
fish fingers or fish cakes	jelly cubes
fish sticks or crab sticks	ice-cream cones
smoked mackerel slices	peanut butter sandwiches
vegetable or soya sausages	muesli bars
vegetable burgers/fingers	marmite on toast
cheese on toast	paté on toast
cheese cubes	vegetable bhajis
fried bean curd cubes	tortilla chips and other large crisps
Jamaican patties	other savoury snacks
kebabs	soft sweets, such as liquorice

(Reproduced with kind permission from 'VOICES').

3(d) Does the person eat food or drink from other people's plates or glasses?

There may be a variety of reasons why a person eats or drinks from someone else's plate or glass. Bathgate *et al* (2001) found in their survey that stealing from others' plates as well as overeating, was more commonly associated with frontotemporal dementia than Alzheimer's disease. In some individuals with Alzheimer's disease, this may relate to the spatial problems discussed under 3(d). The person may not be able to judge distances, and so be unable to tell which glass is theirs. It could relate to the person wanting a certain type of food, or still being hungry – for example, eating their pudding and then taking someone else's. It may be simply that the person has forgotten which bowl is theirs. In these cases, the spacing of residents should be considered, along with simplifying the table. Such difficulties are likely to be worse on a very crowded or busy table. Adequate mealtime help and supervision will help to reduce possible arguments.

3(e) Is the person distracted by other utensils or items on the table?

Some individuals tend to be distracted by items on the table, and instead of ignoring these, stop eating and fiddle with them. For these people, the aim should be to simplify the table as much as possible, by giving them only what they need at that point in the meal, and removing all other utensils, plates or menus. This does not mean the person cannot experience choices when eating. They can be offered a choice, but once they have chosen, all other unnecessary items should be removed. Bayles (1995) advocates that the environment, including mealtimes, should be progressively simplified as the dementia worsens. She refers to this as 'pruning the environment'.

3(f) Is the person messy when eating?

Being messy when eating is caused by a range of factors, including feeding difficulty, postural problems, poor limb control, and behavioural difficulty. Consider if the person has any of the difficulties highlighted under sections 3(b), 3(c) and 3(e). A simpler meal table and better positioning (eg, sitting closer to the table) and supervision are likely to reduce mess. If food is coming off the edge of the plate, a plate guard or bowl should be used. Use napkins on the lap and front to reduce the mess on clothes.

If the person is experiencing behavioural problems, refuses or throws food, consider the issues raised in Section 2. If necessary, ask the doctor to refer them to a community psychiatric nurse or psychiatrist, for advice on behavioural management.

Also consider if their nutritional intake is adequate. It may be that they are so messy that not enough food is being consumed. In such cases you may need to ensure that the food taken is high in calories, and that the person is offered snacks in between meals.

3(g) Does the person mix different courses together?

A common problem in dementia is mixing main course and pudding. While this may be upsetting for relatives and other residents, the person concerned is likely to be unaware of their actions. Remember that while peaches on top of fish may not be socially acceptable, it is fine to have apple sauce on pork: differences are often governed by the social conventions around eating in a given culture, that have been learnt over time. The way to handle this problem is simply to serve courses separately, and not put out the pudding until the person has eaten all they wanted of the main course.

3(h) For those fed by another, are there any concerns regarding the feeder's approach?

For those in the advanced stages of dementia, feeding times are a valuable source of social contact and stimulation. If there is a rush to feed them, then they are being deprived of the full benefit of this contact. Such an atmosphere may be conveyed unintentionally. Feeding should be seen less as a task to complete, and more as a therapeutic activity. Athlin and Norberg (1987b) studied the literature on interaction between the demented person and their caregiver at mealtimes, and proposed a model of care for this area. They argue that not only is the process of interaction important, but also impacting on this is the philosophy of care, the environment, the organisation and the education provided. The caregiver must be sensitive to the person's communication and to subtle cues. Communication becomes more impaired and difficult to decipher as the illness progresses, and increasing reliance needs to be placed on nonverbal reactions, rather than speech. Knowledge of the individual concerned is vital, as well as an understanding of dementia. A philosophy of care that outlines respect for the person and their feelings, needs and wishes is integral to this process.

Although such individuals may not be able to understand the spoken word, they are likely still to be able to pick up a frustrated tone of voice, or sense that the mood is tense. The feeder should sit facing the person and make eye contact when feeding (Kolodny & Malek, 1991). Standing up will encourage the person to look up at the feeder, thus extending their neck and making effective swallowing harder. The feeder should encourage the person by telling them about the food, and giving verbal prompts to chew and swallow as required, as it appears that people with dementia may still respond to such prompts. A calm tone of voice should be used. It may be necessary to be firm, but shouting will only compound problems.

It has been shown that ensuring there is consistency in staff, so that the same staff members work with the same residents, helps them interpret the person's eating behaviours (Athlin & Norberg, 1998). A regular caregiver may be more tuned in to the person's nonverbal communication or signs of difficulty – for example, if the person has not swallowed a mouthful, does not like the taste of the food, or there has been a change in their eating behaviour. As outlined above, some individuals may be able to partially feed themselves. This should be encouraged wherever possible – for example, holding the cup when drinking. The case study of Ralph illustrates this.

Ralph

Ralph had suffered a series of strokes, which caused a vascular dementia and limb weakness on one side of the body. He had a number of problems at mealtimes. He was very easily distracted by any noise or visual stimuli, and was often in a distressed state. He grasped at the feeder – eg, at their hand, arm, or hair – and had a powerful grasp and could not let go easily. At times this led to further verbal or physical aggression. He was fed in his wheelchair, and often slid down in it. Sometimes he did not open his mouth to the food. In addition, the person feeding him would often stand up, and he tried to look up at them while he was eating and drinking, thus extending his neck. He often coughed on his drinks, and occasionally on soft diet.

To help Ralph, he was moved to a quieter area of the dining-room, away from the main door. Calm classical music was played (Ralph had an interest in classical music). This improved his concentration. Following advice from the physiotherapist, he was fed in a chair with more upright support, and his feet could be placed on the ground. The chair had arms and Ralph was encouraged to hold on to the arm of the chair or a small beanbag when being given food, to reduce grasping of the feeder's arms. The feeder sat down facing him when feeding, and prompted him – eg, 'Ralph – open your mouth' when necessary. He was given thickened fluids to drink, and was encouraged to hold the cup for himself, with help. This led to a much calmer approach to mealtimes, with more cooperation from Ralph, and far less coughing after swallowing.

Training staff in feeding techniques, particularly for those with swallowing problems and challenging behaviours, is important. Role play or feeding each other can be useful to give staff a chance to consider how the person may feel in such situations.

4 Assessment and management issues related to food and drink and swallowing

In this section (and Section 5), disorders of swallowing (dysphagia) are considered, as well as food preferences and problems with poor dietary intake. Kayser-Jones (1996) argues that swallowing problems (particularly those of a mild nature) are not always recognised by nursing staff. It is the role of the speech and language therapist, in addition to assessment of such difficulties, to teach other staff to more effectively recognise the signs of swallowing difficulty, and what to do if they occur. Because there are relatively few speech and language therapists working in the field of dementia, many people are not referred for assessment as they should be (Alzheimer's Society, 2000). There is therefore a need for increased training initiatives for staff in this field.

You will find it useful to consult other texts for more detailed information regarding swallowing. The following is a brief summary of the swallowing process, and the effects on it of age and disease, for those who are unfamiliar with this.

Logemann (1983), in her influential text, identified the four phases, once food or drink has reached the mouth, of the swallowing process:

1 Oral preparatory phase

In this first phase, the food is chewed, tasted and mixed with saliva. Lip seal is maintained to prevent food or fluid leaking from the mouth, and the cheek muscles work to prevent significant quantities of food from falling into the sulcus between the jaw and the cheek. Normal breathing is maintained through this phase. The food is then gathered together on to the tongue to form a bolus, the tongue cupping the food against the hard palate.

2 Oral phase

The tongue propels the food backwards against the roof of the mouth in an anterior to posterior rolling action, until the pharyngeal swallow is triggered. The lips remain closed and there is tension in the cheek muscles to facilitate the necessary pressure within the oral cavity.

During the oral phases, sensory information on taste and general sensation are transmitted by cranial nerves V (trigeminal), VII (facial) and IX (glossopharyngeal) (Groher, 1997). Motor information is transmitted via cranial nerves V for chewing, VII for movement of the lips and cheeks, and XII (hypoglossal) for movement of the tongue (Groher, 1997).

The two oral phases are under voluntary control and because of this, in the author's experience, problems tend to emerge initially in these stages in Alzheimer's disease. Feinberg *et al* (1992) found oral stage dysfunction in 71 per cent of a sample of people with advanced dementia. Difficulties with these stages include over-chewing, holding, poor control of the bolus, problems initiating the oral stage of the swallow, and food or fluid escaping from the bolus and trickling into the airway.

3 Pharyngeal phase

This is the swallow reflex. In this phase, the soft palate closes off the nasal cavity and the bolus is directed through the pharynx. The larynx is raised and closed to protect the airway, and the sphincter muscle at the base of the pharynx relaxes to allow the bolus to pass into the oesophagus. The bolus moves through the pharynx via a progressive contractile wave. The stimuli that trigger the pharyngeal swallow have not been defined precisely. However, sensory signals via the cranial nerves are involved in carrying information to the 'swallowing centres' in the medulla within the brain stem. When appropriate incoming signals are received, a motor response is sent via cranial nerves IX, X (vagus) and XII (Groher, 1997). Feinberg *et al*'s (1992) sample found 43 per cent of individuals with advanced dementia had pharyngeal dysfunction. Such difficulties include food and fluid pooling in the valleculae and pyriform sinuses (within the pharynx); defective movement and propulsion of the bolus; defective laryngeal closure, and food and fluid penetrating the airway or being further aspirated into the lungs. Many people with dementia have multiple stage swallowing dysfunction (Feinberg *et al*, 1992 noted 42 per cent).

4 Oesophageal phase

The bolus passes down the oesophagus into the stomach, by gravity and peristalsis.

The effectiveness of the swallow is therefore dependent on coordination of a number of muscles, including the lips, tongue, cheeks, soft palate, pharynx, larynx and muscles of respiration. Muscles are involved in breakdown and movement of the bolus, as well as maintenance of seals – for example, the lips and nasopharnx – and maintenance of pressure in the oral and pharyngeal cavity. Equally important is information generated from sensory stimulation of these areas. This allows the swallow to adjust to different volumes, consistencies, viscosity and temperature of the bolus. Any damage to the relevant cranial nerves, or the areas of the brain controlling and interpreting these motor and sensory functions, may give rise to problems in swallowing.

Hudson *et al* (2000), in a review article, identify that there may be changes to the swallowing mechanism in the normal elderly. For example, research has highlighted decreased salivary flow; increased motor response time needed for chewing and initiating the swallow; changes in coordination of swallowing and breathing, and changes in pharyngeal peristalsis (eg, Tracey *et al*, 1989; Nilsson *et al*, 1996). In addition, there may be sensory changes such as decreased taste and smell, that impact on chewing and swallowing (Rolls, 1989). Researchers speculate that these changes result in a decreased functional reserve. This means that these age-related changes are subtle; they may slow the swallowing process, but they do not interfere greatly with everyday swallowing skills (Ekberg & Feinberg, 1991), and do not cause dysphagia. However, the general health status of an individual is important. In the frail aged individual, decreased physical conditioning may interact with age-related changes. Swallowing may be affected by changes that are secondary to other systemic illness (Cherney, 1994) – for example, an infection may weaken an elderly person and lead to swallowing problems, when no such difficulties have occurred in the past. Hudson *et al* (2000) also highlight that malnutrition may cause weakness, and so impact on swallowing function, thus illustrating the interdependent relationship between dysphagia and malnutrition. In the author's experience, severe depression can lead to symptoms of dysphagia in elderly frail people. This could be due to the effects of poor appetite and oral intake, leading to low energy, fatigue, etc; or it could be due to physical slowing of the motor system, causing incoordination of the swallow.

The most common cause of dysphagia in the elderly is neurological disease, and this can have profound effects on swallowing function. For example, the prevalence of swallowing difficulties after stroke ranges from 25 per cent to 32 per cent (Groher & Bukatman, 1986). In many, this is a temporary problem. Barer (1989) showed that in the survivors of CVA with initial dysphagia, improvement was common within the first week, and of those with persisting impairment at one week, 80 per cent showed improvement at a month. This means that for such individuals, regular review of their swallowing is required. Individuals with vascular dementia may experience problems in swallowing due to each episode of stroke. While some may deteriorate continuously across a range of functions, including swallowing, others may show a more step-wise deterioration, with even an improvement in function between episodes. Therefore a diagnosis of vascular dementia does not necessarily preclude some improvement in the dysphagic symptoms, particularly for those in the earlier stages of the disease. Regular review is required, and it should not be assumed that dietary changes are always permanent.

About 50 per cent of patients with Parkinson's disease have dysphagia, usually as the disease progresses, as a result of both oral/pharyngeal and oesophageal dysfunction (Lieberman *et al*, 1980). Feinberg *et al* (1992) examined the videofluoroscopies of 131 patients with advanced dementia, and found that only 7 per cent had a normal swallow. Those working in the field recognise that dysphagia is a common problem, particularly in those with advanced dementia.

Typical difficulties with swallowing due to neurological disease include:

◆ Poor lip seal with food escaping when eating
◆ Problems chewing food

- Poor bolus preparation
- Difficulty initiating a swallow, with 'holding' of food and fluid, and a delayed swallow
- A weak or incoordinated swallow, leading to pooling of material in the pharynx and aspiration of food into the airway.

Logemann (1983) describes 'aspiration' as the generic term used to refer to the action of material penetrating the larynx and entering the airway below the true vocal folds. This can occur in anyone; however, in an alert person it would usually be followed by a reflex cough to clear the airway. In those with swallowing problems, the reflex cough may also be impaired, causing material to remain in the trachea and bronchial tree. Infiltration of this material into the lungs can lead ultimately to aspiration pneumonia in some people.

At times, a person with swallowing problems may not cough at all, or show any obvious outward sign of difficulty when they aspirate. They are therefore referred to as 'silent aspirators'. This is true of about 40 per cent of dysphagic patients who aspirate (Logemann, 1983). Groher (1997) states that there are several factors associated with a reduced laryngeal cough reflex, including damage to the sensory or motor pathways of the reflex; medications; decreased level of arousal, and cognitive impairment. Therefore, it is extremely important that people are observed closely, and that it is recognised by all staff that, just because a person does not cough, does not mean they do not have any difficulties.

A standard bedside dysphagia assessment usually starts with a detailed examination of the muscles involved in chewing, swallowing and breathing, followed by trying the person on small amounts of various textures, usually starting with fluids. The therapist will feel for a swallow by placing a hand under the person's chin with the fingers spread. The index finger is placed just behind the mandible, the middle finger on the hyoid bone, the third finger at the top of the thyroid cartilage, and the fourth finger at the bottom of the thyroid cartilage (Logemann, 1993).

People with dementia often have difficulty cooperating with such formal procedures, and therefore assessment of these areas may be possible only through observation (Cherney, 1994).

4(a) Does the person experience significant drooling of saliva or food?

With saliva (note lips and jaw at rest) and consistency of saliva (normal/thick), note the following:

As saliva is produced constantly, reduced swallowing may cause it to build up in the oral cavity, leading to drooling. For some people, excessive saliva production may be due to the side effects of medication, so check for this. Some may not be able to safely swallow their own saliva, and may therefore be at risk of aspiration of this. Note if there is reduced tone in the oral musculature, often with mouth breathing, and drooling at rest. Note if the saliva is normal in consistency, or particularly thick and difficult to manage.

With food (note jaw and lip opening, lip protrusion, lip closure and sensation), note the following (Cherney, 1994):

◆ Ability to open jaw and lips to a spoon or cup, and if prompting helps this
◆ Ability to initiate and maintain protrusion for removal of food from the utensil
◆ Ability to close lips around the spoon or cup to retrieve food or fluid
◆ Ability to maintain closure during chewing and swallowing
◆ Leakage of food and fluid
◆ Awareness of food or fluid leakage.

Take note of this performance on different consistencies, to see if altering consistency could enhance performance. Also consider if posture or feeding technique could be improved.

4(b) Are there observable signs of tongue weakness or dysfunction before or during eating?

Reduced range of movement – note difficulty forming or moving the bolus in the oral cavity. This may be due to weakness in the tongue. Occasionally there may be very little or no movement of the bolus, caused by severe oral apraxia, reduced oral sensation, or a lack of recognition of the bolus as food (Logemann, 1998). Logemann (1998) advises an increase in sensory stimulation, by increasing the pressure of the spoon on the tongue, increasing the size of the bolus, or experimenting with different tastes and temperatures – cold, sweet, sour, etc. Note the effects of texture and consistency – some carers anecdotally report better performance on more solid or textured food than puréed food, often occurring when the person has helped themselves to food, or a biscuit, for example. This may be because chewing has been triggered by the texture, and this has then elicited the swallow (Logemann, 1998). In such cases it may be useful to try different textures, carefully, and under supervision.

Tongue thrust – this is an abnormal reflex response (Groher, 1997). Groher states that it is reduced by facilitating tongue retraction, which can be aided by chin tuck or head flexion. Therefore attention to posture is important.

Repetitive movements – note any patterns that emerge. These may be caused by medication (see Chapter 3, question 13), or neurological damage.

Other areas may include:

Tongue pumping – for those people who will allow you to feel on their throat for a swallow, this may be felt under the chin, through the floor of the oral cavity, and is often due to unsuccessful attempts to initiate a swallow.

Sucking – a primitive reflex that may emerge as the higher centres of the brain become damaged. Groher (1997) argues that this may be observed as part of a suck-swallow sequence, and could be used to elicit a reflexive swallow, when a volitional swallow is absent, for nutritional reasons.

Taken together, 4(b) and 4(c) will help you decide if changing consistencies will be helpful.

4(c) Does the person have difficulty chewing or swallowing particular consistencies?

Signs of swallowing problems include poor chewing; holding, rather than swallowing food and fluid; a delayed swallow; coughing or throat clearing after a swallow, or continuous oral movements that interfere with the chewing and swallowing process. Some people may cram food and not chew or swallow adequately, leading to coughing or even choking.

It is important to note the person's ability to swallow on a variety of textures. If necessary, the diet can then be modified to avoid the textures that cause difficulty.

Problems with solids?

People who have poor chewing, or find it hard to move food from the front to the back of the mouth, are likely to have more difficulty with solid food. Note if they chew with a rotary pattern or a vertical chop, or if chewing is absent (Cherney, 1994). If individuals are at risk of aspiration, and the material swallowed is solid food that has not been chewed properly, airway obstruction (choking) may result (Logemann, 1983). A softer diet would be safer for such people. Those who eat very quickly, without chewing properly, and pack their mouths with food, are also likely to have more problems with solids (a pattern often seen in frontotemporal dementia/Picks disease). A softer and more moist diet may also be necessary here, as well as strategies to reduce the speed of eating (see Section 2f).

A soft diet does not necessarily mean a liquidised or puréed diet. There are plenty of normal foods available that are soft, and many people may still be able to manage this texture. Burge (1994) has described the use of textured soft diets for the elderly mentally infirm, rather than resorting to liquidised food. In this diet, food should be soft enough to be mashed with a fork, and all tough or fibrous food removed. Crumbly or sticky food should be avoided, including dry biscuits or white bread that can become sticky in the mouth.

Holding food, or over chewing prior to swallowing, can be difficult symptoms to manage, and are common problems in Alzheimer's disease. Try a softer and more moist diet, and give the person verbal prompts to chew and swallow. There is anecdotal evidence that some people may be more likely to elicit a swallow if they are involved in feeding themselves, rather than being fed. This may be because the life-long pattern of eating begins with the hand moving the food or drink to the mouth. This could be seen as the preliminary stage in a chain of events, each helping to trigger the next event. Therefore, it may be useful to get the person to help you by holding the spoon while you guide it to their mouth. If they continue to hold the food in their mouth, try guiding their hand for the next mouthful, and see if this triggers a swallow. Experiment with different tastes, textures and temperatures, to see if this elicits better recognition of food and therefore a better swallow – for example, a sweet versus a sour bolus (see under 'fluids'), spicy or strong-tasting food, or ice-cream.

Mashed ice chips have been proposed by many authors for people in the terminal stages of a dementia, to maintain comfort.

Occasionally, holding can occur in people who are self-feeding. They may carry on eating although they have not swallowed each mouthful. The author has seen this in a number of people with frontotemporal dementia/Pick's disease. Again, move to a much softer diet, and supervise them at mealtimes, to ensure they do not pack their mouths full, and choke as a result.

Some people may have very severe chewing and swallowing problems, and so be able to manage only a puréed or liquidised diet. If this is the case, ensure that the diet contains enough fibre. Fruit and vegetables can be cooked and easily puréed. Be aware that adding significant amounts of water may reduce the nutritional content of a meal (VOICES, 1998). It is best to purée each part of the meal separately, as this maintains a range of tastes and sensory stimulation.

Finally, remember to pay particular attention to dentition when considering solid food (see Section 1(d).

Problems with bitty or lumpy food?

Some people may find lumpy or bitty foods hard to eat. Such foods are of a mixed texture – for example, some soups, cereal with cold milk, food with skins or pips etc – and are difficult for those with swallowing problems because they have to manage two textures in their mouth at once (VOICES, 1998). If they keep spitting out, coughing or throat clearing on the lumps, move to a softer texture – food with only soft lumps that could be mashed easily. Some people may also cough on crumbly textures, such as crumbly biscuits. Reduced ability to keep the bolus together can result in coughing on the crumbs.

Avoid liquidising all food too early, to maintain chewing if possible.

Problems with fluids?

People with swallowing problems, particularly with a delayed swallow, may have difficulty with swallowing thin fluids. The more fluid a substance is, the more likely it will be aspirated and travel further into the respiratory system. This appears to be due to the simple fact that fluids are likely to travel more quickly, and be harder to control (Logemann, 1983). Poor tongue control of the fluid bolus, for example, could lead to fluids leaking over the back of the tongue and being aspirated before a swallow reflex is triggered effectively. Some may 'hold' fluid prior to a swallow triggering, which may also be aspirated in part. For people who cough, throat clear or appear gargly after swallowing fluids, thickening their drinks with a thickening agent may help. This will slow down the movement of the fluid and give the person more control and time to initiate a swallow. It may also help people who drool significant amounts of fluid out of their mouth when drinking, due to poor lip and tongue tone and movement. Drinks can be thickened to a variety of textures, depending on the severity of the problem. Thickening agents can be obtained on prescription from the person's doctor in Britain and many other countries (or consult the pharmacist).

However, some people may still drool the thickened fluid out of their mouth before it can be swallowed. A cup with an extended lip may help. Cups are also available with a slant or side cut away, so pouring without tipping the head can be managed. You may wish to ask the physiotherapist for advice, if the person's head posture makes drinking difficult for them. For some people with dementia, when they become very unwell they may find drinking from a cup, even with help, very difficult. In such instances, they may need their thickened fluids to be fed to them on a spoon. This can be very time consuming for staff, but may be the only safe and effective way to feed them.

It is often difficult for people with dementia to understand and retain the reasons for thickening fluids, leading to arguments with staff. This can be exacerbated when drinks are too thick, so they are hard to pour and unpalatable. The more normal a drink seems, the more likely it is to be accepted. You may wish to consider thick 'milkshake drinks', or drinks with stronger tastes. For those living at home in the community, ready thickened drinks may be better, and these are now available. They are useful for people living alone, or to reduce the burden on an elderly carer.

As with solids (see explanation above), some people are better if they are more involved in the eating process. Encouraging the person to hold the cup, even if you guide it to their mouth, may reduce holding. If they do not swallow that mouthful, guide their hand and cup gently back to their mouth, but do not give another mouthful, and see if this action helps to trigger a swallow. Again, for those who are 'holding' fluid prior to swallowing, you should try with different temperatures (eg, very cold) or tastes. Some practitioners have tried using either a very sweet bolus (eg, sugar), or a sour bolus (eg, lemon juice or grapefruit juice), to elicit a swallow. Logemann *et al* (1995) found a significant improvement in oral onset of the swallow with a sour, cold bolus (lemon juice) in people with stroke and other neurological diseases. They postulated that the sour bolus serves as a preswallow sensory alert to the nervous system. The Caroline Walker Trust (1995) suggests that older people should drink a minimum of 1.5 litres of fluid each day (equivalent to about 8 to 10 cups). Dehydration can cause headaches, confusion, irritability, constipation, loss of appetite and urinary tract infections, so fluid intake must be carefully monitored (VOICES, 1998).

Remember that changes to a person's diet will need to be reviewed, particularly if there is a change in their condition. For example, a person's swallow may deteriorate due to a stroke, and this may require a modified diet. However, even in a vascular dementia they may recover some function with time, and show improvement in their swallowing. It may then be possible to increase the range of textures the person can eat. Others may deteriorate in a range of functions, including swallowing, due to co-occurring medical conditions, which when treated can result in some improvement. This was true in the case of Mr Smith.

Mr Smith

Mr Smith had vascular dementia. He was normally very passive, but could feed himself slowly with no difficulty. However, he became unwell and developed increasing problems with his mobility. Investigations showed that he had a chest infection. In addition, he became unable to feed himself reliably, and was more confused than usual. He coughed when given thin fluids, and when given solids, he over-chewed repeatedly.

Mr Smith was treated for his chest infection, and he was moved on to thickened fluids with a soft or mashed diet (ie, soft enough to be mashed with a fork, but not liquidised). His general condition improved greatly over the following month or so. He became more alert, and soon was able to feed himself. His swallowing improved, and he was moved back on to thin fluids. Mr Smith was able to eat some softer solids, but continued to have to avoid bread and tough meat.

Staff acted quickly in managing Mr Smith's swallowing problems – eg, reducing the risk of aspiration on thin fluids – and so further complications were prevented. In addition, they monitored his condition, and were able to move him back to a more normal diet when he was able to take it. This shows that a diagnosis of dementia does not necessarily preclude improvement.

4(d) Is there a delay in triggering the swallow?

A delayed swallow, due to difficulty initiating the swallow reflex, is a common problem in those with advanced dementia and swallowing dysfunction. In such people, it may be possible to feel the tongue moving or 'pumping' to try to initiate the swallow. Consider if altering the textures taken would be appropriate – for example if a softer diet would be better, or if the person is at risk of aspiration on thin fluids. See if verbal prompting helps, or in some cases, for example with oral apraxia, indirect cues such as talking about the food may be more helpful – for example, 'that tastes nice' (Logemann, 1998). If difficulties are severe, examine if carefully giving the person the next mouthful (as described above), helps to trigger the event. Wherever possible, involve the person in holding the cup or spoon.

4(e) Is there repeated coughing, throat clearing or choking after swallowing?

If these symptoms occur after swallowing, it is likely that food or fluid has penetrated the airway. In severe instances, food may block the airway and cause choking. In people with brain disease, the cough reflex may be ineffective, leading to repeated throat clearing or what, in some, may even sound like attempted vocalisations. The protective cough mechanism is therefore defective, putting the person at risk of aspiration and its effects. This means that the presence of throat clearing, as well as coughing, should be carefully noted by all staff. Note the effects of consistency on this, and alter texture as appropriate. See if better posture reduces coughing. See under section 3(h) to examine if feeding style or rate is exacerbating the situation.

4(f) Is there a change to a wet, gargly voice quality after swallowing?

This symptom is also suggestive of aspiration of food or fluid into the airway, coupled with an ineffective cough. It is referred to as silent aspiration (Horner & Massy, 1988). In such instances, the cough reflex may be absent, and the only sign that material has entered the airway is when the person vocalises, and the presence of the material can be heard in their voice quality. This is usually assessed by asking the person to vocalise – for example, say 'ah' – before and after swallowing, to note any change in voice quality. People with dementia may find this too abstract, so asking them 'is that nice' and listening for a change in whatever vocalisation you are given, may be the only option. Many individuals may be unable to speak or vocalise spontaneously in such situations, and so listening to breathing before and after swallowing is useful. Breathing that becomes laboured or gargly post swallow, is a concern. Again, examine if a change in food and fluid texture is necessary. Consider thickening fluids.

4(g) Does the person need several swallows to clear each mouthful?

Either watch or feel on the person's neck to see when they elicit a swallow. You may be able to count multiple swallows, taken to clear each mouthful because the person's swallow is inefficient, and residue is left in the oral and pharyngeal cavity. These people may need a slower feeding rate, to allow time for such multiple swallows – a factor of which less experienced staff may not be aware.

4(h) Does the person have difficulty with particular foods – eg, bread or meat – or with swallowing tablets?

Some people with milder swallowing difficulties may have problems, not with a range of textures, but with particular foods. For example, reports of difficulty chewing meat, or bread sticking (white bread in particular) are common. In such cases, it must be made clear to all concerned which foods to avoid. Many people with dementia will not be able to remember why they cannot have something, so it is worth pursuing other palatable options that they can have instead. Being told you cannot have a biscuit at tea time, with everybody else, can be very upsetting if you do not understand why. Being given a soft mousse or other treat that is 'specially for you', may go down better.

Tablets are often the hardest to manage. In some cases this is due to the mixed texture of solid (tablet) and fluid to wash it down. Some people may cough on tablets, or may appear to have swallowed them, but then spit them out later. Check with the person's doctor to ascertain if medications could be prescribed in liquid form. Also check if medication can be crushed, and taken with food, eg jam. This is important, as some tablets are specially coated, or come in capsule form to enable slow release into the system, and should be swallowed whole.

4(i) Is the size of the mouthfuls taken a concern?

People who take mouthfuls that are too large may have lost the judgement to know what is both a manageable, and socially acceptable amount, to put in their mouth at once. They may, for example, try to cram a large potato in their mouth, without recognising that it is impossible to chew. This may make the person cough and choke on their food. Cramming of food has been associated with frontotemporal dementia (Bathgate *et al*, 2001). Such people may also overeat and take food from the plates of others. Combat this by cutting food into small pieces. These people should be supervised and encouraged to swallow each mouthful, either by verbal prompts, or a gentle hand on theirs to stop them eating for a moment, and chew and swallow. Encouragement to put down their knife and fork during the meal for a brief period may also help. Try giving them a smaller utensil – a teaspoon rather than a dessert spoon, for example. If choking occurs regularly, try giving a softer and more moist diet. See 2(f) for advice regarding speed of eating.

People who take very small mouthfuls often eat very slowly, and may take only small amounts of diet. Often food becomes cold and unappetising. Serve each course separately, keeping it hot if possible, or consider using a heat-retaining plate. Record their dietary intake to see if they are taking adequate amounts of diet, and monitor any weight loss. Encourage the person to eat small snacks between meals if weight loss occurs, and ensure the food that they do take is high in calories. Refer those you are concerned about to the dietitian for further advice. If difficulties are severe and the person is not eating enough, they may need to be fed part of their meal – for example, the second half of it, or in some cases all of it.

4(j) Is the temperature of the food or drink too hot, or too cold?

A person with dementia may be unable to gauge the temperature of food. Many authors have reported anecdotally that pain perception may be altered in dementia, and that 'reflex' responses to hot stimuli are diminished. The person may continue to eat very hot food, even if it burns their mouth. They are therefore reliant on others to ensure that their food is served at the right temperature. For slow eaters, however, food may go cold and become unappetising. As described above, courses should be served separately to maintain their temperature (this can be a problem in hospitals where food must be served and eaten within a certain time), and a heat-retaining plate may be useful.

4(k) Does the person leave a large proportion of their meal?

It is important to ascertain if the person is taking enough food to maintain their nutritional status. Malnutrition is common in dementia, and this can lead to increased infection rates and longer hospital admissions (Sandman *et al*, 1987). People at particular risk are those who have difficulty feeding themselves, leave large amounts, eat very slowly, take small mouthfuls, or who keep getting up and leaving the table. For such people, it will be necessary to monitor their dietary intake using food and fluid charts, and to weigh them regularly.

VOICES (1998) recommend that all nursing- and residential-home residents should be weighed on admission, and then at least monthly thereafter, and those with a recent unintended weight loss or gain of 3kg or more should be referred for assessment by a doctor and/or dietitian. All homes should have scales, preferably sitting scales, which should be checked regularly. The dietitian will be able to provide advice on increasing the nutritional value of the person's diet, and on fortified drinks and foods, if necessary. They will also be able to advise if the diet is nutritionally balanced.

Volicer (1998) argues that calorific dietary supplements may be better than tea, coffee or soup, as the latter have low nutrient density. Low fat and low sugar options may be given to everyone in hospital and care homes, because some residents are diabetic or on special diets, or due to a lack of understanding regarding 'healthy eating'. However, for many people who are not diabetic and are losing weight, this is not appropriate. Consider if this is part of the routine. Steele (1997) has highlighted that staff should also make an effort to target management strategies at those with mild to moderate cognitive impairment, rather than concentrating all efforts on those individuals who need to be fed to stave off weight loss.

Suski (1989) found that residents with Alzheimer's disease had their optimal dietary intake at the midday meal when they were at their peak. At an individual level, people may vary as to how much they eat at a given meal, for a variety of reasons. Therefore it will be useful to note down the person's particular habits, and consider why this might be – for example, are they more alert then; do they tire at the end of the day; is this meal sweeter, or is it the effects of medication? As stated below (4(m)) some individuals develop food preferences, particularly for sweet foods. They may eat little of savoury foods, and attention needs to be paid to this. For example, should they have extra helpings of sweet food; can more balanced nutrition be provided through this medium – for example, using sweetened, cooked fruit? If a person eats small amounts at a mealtime, efforts should be made to supplement this with snacks at other times, such as biscuits and sandwiches, or yoghurt or mousse for those on a soft diet. Care staff should be able to offer food and drinks to residents whenever required, and snacks and drinks should be available throughout the day and night (VOICES, 1998).

Consider if the person may be depressed and therefore have a poor appetite (Volicer, 1994). Note if they have other signs of depression, such as low mood, tearfulness, negative content to their conversation, low motivation and disturbed sleep pattern. If these are present, you should discuss this with their doctor (see Chapter 3, question 10). If they often refuse food, see Section 2(f) above. It may also be that such individuals require more encouragement to eat, and it is important to note if verbal encouragement, physical prompting and touch (Eaton *et al*, 1986) are provided at mealtimes.

4(l) Does the person have any food and drink preferences or dislikes?

Loss of taste and smell, leading to changes in appetite and food choice, can occur with advancing age, from certain medications, and various disease states including dementia (Schiffman & Graham, 2000). It is well documented that a significant number of people with dementia show an alteration in their food choice (Morris, 1989), and many appear to develop a particular preference for sweet foods (eg, Mungas *et al*, 1990). There are numerous theories as to why this occurs, including imbalance of chemicals in the brain as a result of the disease process; abnormal insulin response, or a form of disinhibited behaviour. Miller *et al* (1995) found that weight gain and sweet and carbohydrate craving was a far more common early symptom in people with frontal lobe dementia than those with Alzheimer's disease. Neary *et al* (1998) list overeating, bingeing, altered food preferences and food fads, along with oral exploration of objects, as one of the supportive features in their classification of the features of frontotemporal dementia. Further research by this team – Bathgate *et al* (2001) showed that people with frontotemporal dementia were more likely than those with Alzheimer's disease to show an altered preference for sweet things and overeating. Keene and Hope (1998), however, noted that overeating did occur in some individuals with Alzheimer's disease. They found that a significant proportion of people went through a stage of overeating, and that this was associated with a change in food preference (especially an increase in sweet food intake), as well as eating non-food items.

It may be that previous likes or dislikes no longer hold true for the person. However, it is worth examining both past and current likes and dislikes, and those of current relevance should be listed clearly in their care plan. If the person has to avoid certain food textures, ascertain whether their likes can still be accommodated – for example, if they like chocolate, but cannot eat solids, try chocolate mousse. Kayser-Jones (1996) advocates that more account should be taken of people's cultural needs and previous preferences, and this may well be a factor in at least some cases of food refusals. The Alzheimer's Society UK (2000) found in their survey that many carers felt individual likes and dislikes were not always taken into account, and that individuals with dementia were often not given enough choice of food in care homes. One of their recommendations is that care homes should reflect the ethnic and cultural diversity of their residents in the provision of daily menus and celebratory meal.

Schiffman and Graham (2000) have suggested that compensating for taste and smell loss with flavour-enhanced food may improve palatability and/or intake in elderly people. This may be worth exploring in people with dementia.

4(m) Is food left in the person's mouth or cheeks at the end of a meal?

Those with swallowing problems may squirrel food in their cheeks, or on the roof of their mouth, at the end of a meal. This is often due to reduced muscle tone, and/or lack of oral sensation. Note if this tends to occur in the same location, eg, left cheek. It is important that these people are given mouth care at the end of each meal, as they are unlikely to be aware that food is there, and are at risk of breathing it in later, particularly if they lie down.

Assessment and management issues related to severe swallowing problems

5 Signs indicative of swallowing problems and possible aspiration

Section 4 outlined the swallowing process. This section discusses the medical and ethical issues raised when people have severe swallowing problems. These are considered in a separate section, to highlight the difficulties in management that such problems present in this group of people.

5(a) Is further investigation of the swallow required – eg, videofluoroscopy?

In some cases, people with swallowing problems will need further investigation, for instance, by a videofluoroscopy of their swallow. This is a 'modified barium swallow', which produces a moving x-ray of a person's swallowing skills, and can identify possible aspiration more objectively. During this procedure, the person can also be given different textures, and the effectiveness of their swallow monitored on each texture to reveal if certain textures, or methods of feeding, reduce the rate of aspiration. It is often assumed that this procedure is not appropriate for people with dementia because they will not be able to cooperate, or it will not change management in any way. However, the author would argue that it is useful in some cases, particularly for those with mild to moderate dementia, and that with time and explanation, such people are able to engage in the procedure. Feinberg *et al* (1992) advocate for more use to be made of the technique with this group. They noted in their study that it did change management in a significant number of cases (28 out of the 131 studied), and that lack of cooperation led to the procedure being discontinued in a small proportion of cases (13 out of the original 144).

5(b) Does the person have severe swallowing problems across all textures?

In people with severe swallowing impairment, significant aspiration may occur across all textures. In some cases, this may lead to repeated chest infections. If this occurs, the medical team will need to decide, in conjunction with the person's family, if they are to continue with oral feeding, or use non-oral methods – ie, tube feeding. The two main types of tube feeding are nasogastric (a tube sited via the nasal cavity through the pharynx, oesophagus and into the stomach) and percutaneous endoscopic gastrostomy, or PEG (a tube sited by medical procedure through the stomach wall directly into the stomach). Such tubes are considered for people with severe swallowing problems and risk of aspiration; those who have a poor swallow and are unlikley to maintain their nutrional status, and those who are severely malnourished. Tube feeding is therefore intended to reduce aspiration of food and drink into the lungs, by bypassing the swallowing system and delivering it straight to the stomach, and/or enable greater amounts of diet to be taken to maintain nutrition and weight. Hydration can be achieved via intravenous or subcutaneous methods, with solutions administered through a catheter inserted into a peripheral vein or subcutaneous tissue. Such procedures may be carried out by medical or nursing staff.

The use of tube-feeding in people with advanced dementia remains controversial, raising medical and ethical questions. Sheiman (1996) comments that the debate in this area often raises questions:

1   Is tube feeding a food or medical treatment?

2   Does it improve quality of life, or does it prolong the dying process?

3   Under what circumstances can tube feeding be withheld, or withdrawn?

The following discussion focuses predominantly on the situation in England and Wales with regard to tube-feeding people with dementia. However, practitioners are advised to find out about the laws (for example, surrounding consent) and medical guidelines regarding this in their own country or state.

The British Medical Association (BMA) has produced a document *Withholding and Withdrawing Life-prolonging Medical Treatment – Guidance for Decision Making* (1999) that discusses the current medical and legal framework in England and Wales for decision-making in this area. This document states that the BMA does not feel it is an appropriate goal of medicine to prolong life at all costs, with no regard to its quality, or the burden of treatment. Following legal judgements, the BMA notes that artificial nutrition and hydration is now considered a medical treatment in English common law, and may be withheld or withdrawn in some circumstances. The association advocates that the benefits, risks and burdens of the treatment in each case should be fully assessed.

The British Association for Parental and Enteral Nutrition (BAPEN, 1999), has also examined the ethical and legal aspects to clinical hydration and nutritional support. It highlights that it is the duty of professionals to prolong life, but not to prolong death inappropriately. The difficulty they say is to define life, and recognise when death is occurring.

The BMA advocates that thorough assessment of the patient should be carried out by the multi-disciplinary team, and any decisions should be based on the best available clinical evidence. It is the role of the speech and language therapist to describe the problem to the medical team, and to the person/carers in an understandable way. The therapist can give advice, but it is not their role to take management decisions of this nature.

The BMA states that competent adults should have their treatment discussed with them, and have the right to refuse any medical treatment, even if that refusal results in their death. In the case of dementia, it should be ascertained if the person is competent or not to make such decisions. Competency is task-specific, and therefore a diagnosis of dementia does not necessarily preclude competency – for example, mildly impaired individuals may be able to make such decisions. For those with communication difficulties, the advice of a speech and language therapist may be useful to ascertain ways to help the person understand, and express their views. However, in more advanced dementia, the person is usually unable to engage in any meaningful communication, or reasoning process, and is therefore not competent. Currently (2002) in English law, it is the person's doctor, with advice from the rest of the healthcare team, who is ultimately responsible for deciding whether treatment is provided without consent. The next of kin therefore have no legal power to give, or withhold consent, contrary to popular belief. However, the BMA advocates that the next of kin should be involved in the consultation process, providing valuable insight into the person's past wishes, values and preferences. Relatives are not being asked to state their own personal wishes, but to discuss what they think would be in the best interest of the person concerned.

The BMA advises that the doctor should also take note of advance directives regarding treatment, as although there is currently no statute on these, a number of legal cases have established their legal weight in England. Good communication with all those involved – ie, person concerned, relatives, friends and professionals – is seen as essential to decision-making.

Tube-feeding may be withheld if the perceived burden exceeds the probable benefit, or if it appears futile (BAPEN, 1999). Tube-feeding may be given if the benefit is judged to outweigh the burden.

This process should be documented carefully in the person's medical notes. All disciplines involved should ensure they keep accurate, up-to-date records of their involvement. Any treatment decisions should be reviewed on a regular basis, both before and after implementation. Should a treatment be instigated, but prove to be of no benefit, or cause excessive burden, the BMA argues that it is not in the person's best interests that this be continued.

BAPEN (1999) notes that with regard to fluids, consideration should be given as to whether the aim of care is to prolong life – for example, to overcome an acute illness caused by infection or the side effects of medication – or to provide comfort. They also state that drinking physiological amounts does not always appear necessary for comfort in the last stages of life. A dry mouth may be a problem, but this can be reduced by sips of water, ice chips, regular mouth care, etc. In this situation they state that 'enforced' drinking is unnecessary and intrusive.

The BMA document has been criticised by some as morally, or religiously wrong – such people arguing that it amounts to euthanasia. However, Gillick (2000) discusses the view that, although people may hold religious values that favour any intervention that offers a chance, no matter how small, of prolonging life, this position is not absolute. In the USA, for example, the Roman Catholic Church's position has been outlined as, 'there should be a presumption in favour of providing nutrition and hydration to all patients, including patients who require medically assisted nutrition and hydration'. This approach is warranted as long as it 'is of sufficient benefit to outweigh the burdens involved to the patient' (National Conference of Catholic Bishops, 1995). The Orthodox Jewish tradition rejects interventions that cause or prolong suffering (Rosin, 1998), and some have argued against impediment to dying, in the last year of life (Schostak, 1994).

Further research and local guidelines in this area are required, but some authors are questioning the medical assumptions behind tube-feeding individuals with advanced dementia, eg, Gillick (2000) and Finucane *et al* (1999). For example, tube feeding is often used to try to reduce the risk of aspiration. However, Peck *et al* (1990) retrospectively examined a group of 52 patients fed by tube against a randomly selected control group fed orally, and found the incidence of aspiration pneumonia to be higher in those who were tube-fed (58 per cent) as compared with those who were not (17 per cent). Gillick (2000) argues that the continued risk of aspiration with tube-feeding may result from the reflux of gastric contents and aspiration of saliva. It has been suggested that tube-feeding can prolong an individual's life; however, Mitchell *et al* (1997) followed up over time a large number of nursing-home residents with severe cognitive impairment, and found survival rates did not differ between groups of residents with and without feeding tubes. They conclude strongly that there are specific risk factors associated with feeding-tube placement in such individuals, and that there are no survival benefits. Volicer *et al* (1989) found that patients with Alzheimer's disease who refused food, or choked on food and fluid, had similar mortality rates to others who did not.

Tube-feeding may be used to try to prevent the consequences of malnutrition. Henderson *et al* (1998) studied 40 people in long-term care, most with neurological impairment, who were tube fed. Despite this method of feeding, subjects continued to show weight loss. Logemann (2000) has suggested that because there may be a malabsorption problem in advanced Alzheimer's disease, tube-feeding may not be appropriate, and argues there is no role for the speech and language therapist at this stage. The author would counter this by suggesting that, while there is evidence for the malabsorption theory, there is still a role for assessment and advice aimed at maintaining optimum feeding strategies, alongside providing support and information to carers at this difficult time. Another reason often cited for tube-feeding is that it reduces pressure sores. Peck *et al* (1990) found in their sample that the reverse was true. Ackerman (1996) argues that we need better controlled research studies to answer these questions. There are, for example, no randomised studies to compare the risk of aspiration with and without tube-feeding in advanced dementia (Gillick, 2000), and in many retrospective studies the tube-fed group may actually be more severely impaired in terms of swallowing function or overall physical health.

Other considerations that reflect burden include whether the person would pull out the tube or need any restraints, physical or pharmacological, should they do so. Despite advanced dementia, many still enjoy eating, and tube-feeding would deprive them of this pleasure. It should be discussed and agreed whether the person is to be kept totally nil by mouth, or if it is possible and safe, to also give them diet – eg, small amounts as 'treats'.

This debate generates radically different views. Some argue that tube-feeding merely prolongs an individual's suffering and death, with very little real quality of life, and that the difficulties in eating presented are the natural end course of dementia. Such authors believe that a more 'hospice' style approach to care is required. For example, Sheiman (1996) comments on the use of glycerine swabs, ice chips (to relieve feelings of dehydration), and improved positioning, communication, companionship, and support with activities of daily living, in the terminal stages of a dementia. Improved pain control is also central to this process.

However, it could also be argued that there is little quality to eating and drinking if the person coughs and chokes on each mouthful, and that for these individuals mealtimes can actually be very distressing. The BMA (1999) states that food and water 'should not be forced upon patients for whom the process of feeding produces an unacceptable level of burden, such as where it causes unavoidable choking or aspiration of the food or fluid'. In clinical practice, some of these individuals, and others, appear to benefit significantly from tube-feeding.

Others believe strongly that life should be preserved at all costs, and that we have no right to withhold food and fluid, even if it needs to be delivered through a tube. They argue that we are unable, and have no right, to judge the quality of another's life, and we should aim to treat them as actively as we can, at all times.

You should think carefully about your views on this topic, and remember that they may not be the same as the families', or as the views previously held by the person with dementia.

Whatever the final decision, the family are likely to need support at such difficult times. Ensuring they are involved, informed and given time to discuss their feeling and concerns, will help them both now and in the future. Nursing staff are well placed to offer ongoing support and advice.

On a final note, it is worth highlighting strongly that the literature in this area tends to concentrate on tube-feeding patients with advanced dementia, as it is often assumed that swallowing problems always occur at the end stage of a dementia. This may be the case in Alzheimer's disease, but some people with other types of dementia – for example, those with vascular dementia – may experience significant swallowing problems at a much earlier stage in the course of an illness. The benefits and burdens may be very different in a less impaired individual, and they may be more likely to benefit from tube-feeding. Assessment of competency to consent is again vital.

The only rule that can be applied in this area is that each case should be considered carefully on its own merits (BMA, 1999; Groher, 1990).

In summary, if tube-feeding is being discussed for an individual, the following points should be covered:

1   What is the aim or benefit of tube-feeding? For example:
   ◆   Will it reduce aspiration?
   ◆   Will it improve nutritional intake?
   ◆   Will it have other positive effects on the person's health, or psychological wellbeing?
   ◆   Will it reduce distress experienced at mealtimes?

2   What are the burdens or drawbacks of tube-feeding? For example:
   ◆   Is the procedure going to pose any risks to the person's health?
   ◆   Will going into hospital/having the procedure, be distressing for them?
   ◆   Will they need any restraints, either physical or pharmacological, to stop them pulling out the tube?
   ◆   Will they miss the pleasure of eating, including the social contact?
   ◆   Will having a tube affect their aftercare or placement – for example, if they are in residential care, is the home willing to accept them with a tube, or will they need to move to a nursing home?
   ◆   Will it have any other negative effects on their health, or psychological wellbeing?

3   Are they to be kept totally nil by mouth if they are to be tube fed, or are they allowed to take any food or fluid orally?

This may be different with people who are given tubes for nutritional reasons, rather than due to aspiration. In the former group, combined oral and tube-feeding may occur, and it is advisable to consult with the dietitian about this. In those who are at risk of aspiration, the team needs to consider if, for example, 'treats' of semi-solids or thickened fluids are appropriate.

4   Is the person competent to take this decision?

5   If they are not competent:
   ◆   Is there an advanced directive?
   ◆   What is known about their prior wishes? (eg, by asking relatives or other professionals involved)
   ◆   Are there any cultural or religious factors that affect decision-making?
   ◆   Has the family been fully consulted?
   ◆   Has the multi-disciplinary team been involved in discussions?

Taking account of all these factors and views, the doctor may then make a decision that is thought to be in the person's 'best interests'.

6   If tube-feeding is initiated, then what goals have been set to measure effectiveness?

7   Has a review date been set to examine these goals?

8   If tube-feeding is not initiated, then is there a clear management plan outlined to manage eating, drinking, and the overall comfort of the person concerned? For example:
   ◆   What consistencies can they be given?
   ◆   Feeding strategies should be outlined
   ◆   Pain relief should be considered
   ◆   What other treatment is necessary?

9   Have goals been set to measure the effectiveness of this plan?

10   Has a review date been set to examine these goals?

11   Have the person and relatives been given adequate information and support, and been involved in discussions throughout this process?

12   Have the effects on staff been considered, and managed, appropriately?

Staff in long-stay environments often have strong emotional ties to residents, which should not be ignored. If oral feeding is to be continued in a person who coughs a great deal, or is hard to feed, this can be distressing for staff involved. Often lower grades of staff carry out feeding, and may not have been involved in the above process. Therefore, training and information are important to all staff.

5

Assessment Profiles

Assessment of feeding and swallowing difficulties in dementia

There are two assessment formats – Format A for less experienced therapists, and Format B for those who are more experienced in this area. Each format covers the same areas.

The assessment is divided into two sections:

◆ **Section 1** History of feeding or swallowing problem

◆ **Section 2** Mealtime observation schedule, which is divided into the following:
Part 1 – Sensory impairment and dentition
Part 2 – Mental state and behaviour
Part 3 – Feeding situation and skills
Part 4 – Issues related to food and drink, and swallowing
Part 5 – Presence of severe swallowing problems.

The literature with respect to each of these areas has been discussed in Chapters 3 and 4. Within the observation schedule, there is overlap between each area, due to the complex nature of eating difficulties in dementia – eg, behavioural disturbance affects a person's ability to feed themselves, and at times, their ability to swallow safely. In addition, the division into 'feeding' and 'swallowing' problems may not be as clear as it first seems – eg, individuals who eat too quickly and take large mouthfuls may cough and choke as a result. Poor feeding technique, and poor positioning of the person, can increase swallowing difficulties.

The history section should be completed by discussion with professionals and carers who know the person, as well as consultation with any medical, psychiatric or nursing records.

To complete the mealtime observation schedule, it is advisable to observe the person, and the mealtime routine, as it usually occurs. Do not feed the person yourself. You may need to observe on more than one mealtime, as problems presented are often variable. It is suggested that you observe different meals – eg, breakfast and evening meal – to see if there are any differences in the person's difficulties at different times of day. Use the questions provided to structure your observations. Space is provided to write down key words or brief notes. It is useful to discuss any observations with others – eg, staff or relatives – to gather further information on these behaviours. If the answer to a question is 'yes', you have highlighted an area of difficulty, and the next task is to provide appropriate management for this. Consult the relevant sections in Chapters 3 and 4, for further information. Advice is presented in checklist form in Chapter 6.

The management advice should be used to construct a care plan to manage the problem. Ensure that all involved at mealtimes, including relatives, are aware of the strategies that should be used. Consistency of approach is vital. The assessment is also designed to highlight those who need to be referred to other disciplines, such as the occupational therapist, dietitian, psychiatric nurse, or doctor.

The assessment should take 20 minutes, on average, to gather the history, and then usually 30 minutes at most, to complete parts 1–5 of the observation schedule.

Assessment Profile – Format A

Name _____ DOB _____

Address _____

_____

Family/carers involved _____ Doctor _____

_____ Professionals involved _____

_____ _____

Assessment carried out by _____

History given by _____

Dates seen			
Time of day			
Setting (where)			

History of feeding/swallowing problem

Past medical and psychiatric history (eg, type of dementia, any repeated chest infections, etc)

_____

_____

_____

_____

_____

_____

_____

_____

1   **When** did the eating/swallowing problem first start?

_____

2   Did it start **gradually/suddenly**?

_____

If the answer to any of the following questions is 'yes' please consult Chapter 3 for further information and advice:

3   Is the problem **getting worse**? Is this gradual or rapid?

_____

4   Has the person experienced repeated **chest infections** in the past year?

_____

5   Has the person lost or gained **weigh**t? Note weight now and 3, 6 and 12 months ago (and before if possible).

_____

6   Are they **diabetic**? How is this controlled and monitored?

_____

7   Is the eating/swallowing problem **variable** from day to day, within the day, or within the meal?

_____

8   Has there been a change in the person's level of **consciousness** and **attention** recently?

_____

9   Has there been a change in the person's **physical health** recently?

_____

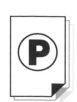

10 Has there been a change in the person's **mood** recently, eg, low in mood?

_____

11 Have there been changes in the person's **behaviour**, eg, disturbed or psychotic behaviour?

_____

12 Does the person complain or nonverbally indicate any **pain** or **discomfort** while eating?

_____

13(a) List the person's current **medication**:

Name of drug	Dose and time	Commenced on
_____	_____	_____
_____	_____	_____
_____	_____	_____
_____	_____	_____
_____	_____	_____

13(b) Do any of these medications have any **side effects** that could affect movement, level of consciousness, concentration, appetite, saliva production, mood or level of confusion?

_____

13(c) Did the eating/swallowing problem occur after a **change** in **medication**?

_____

Mealtime observation schedule Format A

1 SENSORY IMPAIRMENT AND DENTITION	Yes
1(a) Does the person have **visual** difficulties, eg, need glasses or have problems with the ones they have, or have cataract, hemianopia or visual neglect?	
1(b) Does the person need a **hearing** aid, or is the one they have not working?	
1(c) Does the person have problems with **dentition,** eg, need dentures or have problems with their dentures, have infected teeth, poor oral hygiene, or a sore mouth?	

2 MENTAL STATE AND BEHAVIOUR	Yes
2(a) Does the person have a reduced level of **consciousness** (ie, drowsy)?	
2(b) Is it difficult to get the person to **sit for any length** of time at the table?	
2(c) Does the person **forget** what they are doing/become **distracted** from the task?	
2(d) Is the person very **passive**, ie, do they need **prompts** to start eating?	
2(e) Does the person **refuse** food/drink, eg, verbally refuse, push food or feeder away, keep mouth shut, turn head away, spit food out, hit out, etc?	

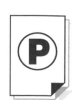

2 MENTAL STATE AND BEHAVIOUR (continued)	Yes
2(f) Is the **speed** of eating/drinking inappropriate, eg, too fast/too slow?	
2(g) Does the person **eat non-food** items?	

3 FEEDING SITUATION AND SKILLS	Yes
3(a) Is the level of mealtime **supervision** inadequate?	
3(b) Is there a problem with the person's **position** when eating, eg, not fully upright, or table/chair not the correct height?	
3(c) Does the person have difficulty **self-feeding**, eg, problems using or locating utensils or crockery on the table?	
3(d) Does the person **eat** food/drink **from others' plates** or glasses?	
3(e) Is the person **distracted** by other utensils or items on the table?	
3(f) Is the person **messy** when eating?	
3(g) Does the person **mix** different **courses** together?	

3 FEEDING SITUATION AND SKILLS (continued)	Yes

3(h) For those fed by another, are there any concerns regarding the **feeder's approach**?

Does it appear overbearing or forceful? _____

Is their tone of voice tense/harsh? _____

Is there a lack of encouragement? _____

Do they appear rushed? _____

Is the feeder standing up, or out of the person's view? _____

4 ISSUES RELATED TO FOOD AND DRINK, AND SWALLOWING	Yes

4(a) Does the person experience significant **drooling** of saliva or food?

Saliva (note lips and jaw at rest) _____

Consistency of saliva (normal/thick?) _____

Drooling food (note jaw and lip opening, lip protrusion, lip closure
and sensation)

_____

4(b) Are there observable signs of **tongue weakness/dysfunction** before or
during eating?

Reduced range of movement _____

Tongue thrust _____

Repetitive movements _____

Other _____

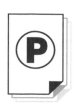

4 ISSUES RELATED TO FOOD AND DRINK, AND SWALLOWING (cont)	Yes
4(c) Does the person have difficulty chewing or swallowing particular **consistencies**? eg, problems chewing, holding food rather than swallowing, coughing/throat clearing post swallow, or continuous oral movements? Solids _____ _____ Bitty or lumpy foods _____ _____ Fluids _____ _____	
4(d) Is there a **delay** in triggering the **swallow**? (Note the effects of consistency on this) _____	
4(e) Is there repeated **coughing, choking or throat-clearing** after swallowing? (Note the effects of consistency on this) _____	
4(f) Is there a change to a **wet, gargly voice** quality after swallowing? (Note the effects of consistency) _____	
4(g) Does the person need **several swallows** to clear each mouthful? (Note the effects of consistency) _____	
4(h) Does the person have difficulty with **particular foods**, eg bread or meat, or with swallowing tablets? _____	
4(i) Is the **size of mouthfuls** taken a concern? Too large _____ Too small _____	

4 ISSUES RELATED TO FOOD AND DRINK, AND SWALLOWING (cont)	Yes
4(j) Is the **temperature of food/drink** too hot or too cold?	
4(k) Does the person **leave a large proportion** of their meal?	
4(l) Does the person have any food **preferences/dislikes**?	
4(m) Is **food left** in the person's **mouth** or cheeks at the end of a meal?	

5 SEVERE SWALLOWING PROBLEMS	Yes
5(a) Is **further investigation** of their swallowing required, eg, videofluoroscopy?	
5(b) Does the person have **severe swallowing problems** across all textures?	

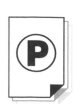

Assessment Profile – Format B

Name _____ DOB _____

Address _____

_____

Family/carers involved _____ Doctor _____

_____ Professionals involved _____

_____

Assessment carried out by _____

History given by _____

Dates seen			
Time of day			
Setting (where)			

History of feeding/swallowing problem

Past medical and psychiatric history (eg, type of dementia, any repeated chest infections, etc)

_____

_____

_____

_____

_____

_____

_____

_____

1   When problem started _____

2   Onset – gradual/sudden _____

3   Progression – gradual/rapid _____

4   Chest infections _____

5   Weight loss/gain _____

6   Diabetic (and how controlled) _____

7   Variability – day-to-day – within day – within meal _____

8   Change in consciousness level/attention _____

9   Physical health _____

10 Mood _____

11 Behavioural disturbance/psychosis _____

12 Pain/discomfort on swallowing _____

13 Medications (a) list (b) note side effects (c) recent changes to medication

_____

_____

_____

_____

_____

_____

_____

_____

Mealtime observation schedule Format B

1 SENSORY IMPAIRMENT AND DENTITION	Yes
1(a) Vision _____	
1(b) Hearing _____	
1(c) Dentition _____	

2 MENTAL STATE AND BEHAVIOUR	Yes
2(a) Consciousness level _____	
2(b) Restless/agitated _____	
2(c) Losing track/distractible _____	
2(d) Passive (needs prompts) _____	
2(e) Refusals _____ _____	
2(f) Speed of eating _____	
2(g) Eating non-food _____	

3 FEEDING SITUATION AND SKILLS	Yes
3(a) Level of supervision _____	
3(b) Positioning _____	
3(c) Self-feeding skills _____	
3(d) Taking food from others _____	
3(e) Distracted by items on table _____	

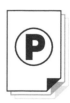

3 FEEDING SITUATION AND SKILLS (continued)	Yes
3(f) Messy _____	
3(g) Mixing courses _____	
3(h) Feeder's approach _____	

4 ISSUES RELATED TO FOOD AND DRINK, AND SWALLOWING	Yes
4(a) Drooling – saliva/food – saliva consistency – lip function _____ _____	
4(b) Tongue – weakness – reduced range – thrust – repetitive movements – other _____	
4(c) Problem consistencies (note chewing, holding, coughing, gargly voice, etc): Solids _____ Bitty/lumpy foods _____ Fluids _____	
4(d) Delayed swallow _____	
4(e) Coughing – throat-clearing – choking – other _____ _____	
4(f) Wet, gargly voice _____	
4(g) Multiple swallows _____	
4(h) Problems with certain foods/tablets _____	
4(i) Size of mouthfuls _____	
4(j) Temperature of food _____	

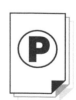

4 ISSUES RELATED TO FOOD AND DRINK, AND SWALLOWING (cont)	Yes
4(k) Leaving food _____	
4(l) Likes/dislikes _____ _____	
4(m) Pouching/oral residue _____	

5 SEVERE SWALLOWING PROBLEMS	Yes
5(a) Further investigation, eg, VF _____	
5(b) Severe problems across all textures _____	

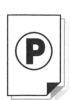

Management Strategies – Checklists

Developing Strategies

You will now have completed the assessment process. Where you have uncovered difficulties, Chapter 4 will highlight the relevant literature in relation to both assessment and management in this area. The task now is to use this information to develop appropriate strategies to help the person with dementia. In some cases you may need to refer to other disciplines; in other cases you will be required to instigate changes in mealtime prompting, feeding, food texture, etc. The latter strategies need to be written into a clear care plan that can be followed by all those involved in the person's care at mealtimes. It is important that the care plan is communicated to everybody, including visiting relatives and friends, in the case of people in hospital or residential care.

Your knowledge of the person and their environment, and discussion with those involved in the person's care, should help you decide which strategies are appropriate. Difficulties presented are complex and individual, so it is impossible to be prescriptive. Therefore it is advisable to instigate any necessary changes in management, and to review their success on a regular basis. If they are unsuccessful, you will need to reassess the situation. Because of the progressive nature of dementia, difficulties presented will change over time, and so will management. Again, regular review is required.

The following checklists are designed to bring together the possible management options.

Tick if needed	1 SENSORY IMPAIRMENT AND DENTITION
	1(a) Does the person have visual difficulties? For example, do they need glasses or have problems with the ones they have, or have cataract, hemianopia or visual neglect? Refer to any medical/psychiatric/therapy/nursing reports for further information on this Check that the glasses used are the correct pair, ie, distance glasses Ensure glasses fit, do not slide down the nose, and are clean Ensure all involved are aware of the need for glasses ***Cataract*** ◆ Discuss this with their doctor ◆ Consider a referral to the local eye hospital/clinic ***Neglect/hemianopia*** ◆ Feeder and food should be placed on their good side ◆ The plate should be turned during the meal Use appropriate verbal and physical prompting during the meal Refer to the optician Refer to occupational therapy for advice on feeding aids for the visually impaired
	1(b) Does the person need a hearing aid, or is the one they have not working? Check the hearing aid is on and working ◆ Change the battery if necessary ◆ Ensure the mould is clear of wax ◆ Check it is on the correct setting If the hearing aid is broken, contact the local audiology clinic

Tick if needed	1 SENSORY IMPAIRMENT AND DENTITION (continued)
	1(b) (continued) Ensure all are aware of the need for the hearing aid Advice should be given for managing hearing loss and communication Ask the doctor to check for impacted wax, or to refer to ENT/Audiology if the person needs a hearing aid or reassessment
	1(c) Does the person have problems with dentition, eg, need dentures or have problems with their dentures, have infected teeth, poor oral hygiene or a sore mouth? Consider the use of denture fixative for loose dentures Give advice on appropriate food textures Regular mouth care or prompting with oral hygiene will be needed Refer to the dentist

Tick if needed	2 MENTAL STATE AND BEHAVIOUR
	2(a) **Does the person have a reduced level of consciousness (are they drowsy)?** Check that the person has been investigated for physical illness, eg, urinary or chest infection, CVA, etc, which may lead to drowsiness and an 'acute confusional state' Check the side effects of medication, and if necessary liaise with their doctor Feed only when alert enough to swallow safely Ensure food is high in calories if small amounts of diet are taken Document the need for mouth care after each meal/snack If you are concerned, ask the doctor to review them
	2(b) **Is it difficult to get the person to sit for any length of time at the table?** Consider possible strategies for this, eg: ◆ Let the person wander until food has arrived ◆ Use simple verbal prompting/show them the food to aid understanding ◆ Give extra helpings when the person is more settled ◆ Include advice from section 2(c) Check if agitation could be a side effect of their medication Consider the use of finger foods that they can consume while on the move

Tick if needed	2 MENTAL STATE AND BEHAVIOUR (continued)
	2(c) Does the person forget what they are doing, or become distracted from the task? Consider possible strategies for this: ◆ Take them to the toilet before the meal ◆ Use verbal prompts to keep them on track ◆ Use gentle physical prompts, eg put utensil/cup back in the person's hands ◆ Gently guide them back to the table and prompt them to continue Reduce environmental distractions Foster a calming environment, eg, calming background music
	2(d) Is the person very passive, ie, do they need prompts to start eating? Consider possible strategies for this: ◆ Draw the person's attention to the food, eg, talk about it ◆ Put the utensil in their hand or guide them to take the first mouthful ◆ If necessary, feed the first mouthful and then try to encourage self-feeding ◆ Give verbal and physical prompts during the meal to continue ◆ Give verbal and physical prompts to move from one course on to the next Consider if it would help them to sit with more able residents they could copy, or be prompted by Check for signs of depression As a last resort only, they may need to be fed part or all of their meal

Tick if needed	2 MENTAL STATE AND BEHAVIOUR (continued)
	2(e) Does the person refuse food/drink?

2(e)   Does the person refuse food/drink?

Advise staff to record or chart the person's exact behaviour in detail, eg, over a week including:

◆ Any verbalisations/nonverbal behaviour

◆ Mood at the time

◆ Time of day

◆ Food/drink and its texture (eg, solids, semisolids, etc)

◆ Wider environment, eg, noise level

◆ Any successful strategies

Consult with staff and relatives to elicit any patterns; adjust management

Check feeding technique/approach, and adjust if necessary (see 3(i))

Coax person to try first mouthful to get 'taste'; use indirect prompts, 'that's nice'

Assess if the person more readily opens their mouth to a spoon or drink – eg, if opening their mouth to a cup occurs more readily than to a spoon, try with a few mouthfuls of fluid first, then move on to the spoon; others may have the reverse pattern. Involve them in self-feeding as much as possible

If they leave a large proportion of their meal see Section 4(e)

Check for delayed swallow, and if this occurs, advise feeding at a slower rate

Experiment with different tastes and textures

Monitor for signs of depression and seek medical advice if necessary

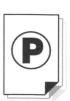

*Feeding & Swallowing
Disorders in Dementia*
© Jackie Kindell 2002
You may photocopy
this page for
instructional use only

Tick if needed	2 MENTAL STATE AND BEHAVIOUR (continued)
	2(f) Is the speed of eating or drinking inappropriate?

Too fast

Consider possible strategies for this:

- Cut food into small pieces
- Supervise to slow down with verbal and physical prompts
- Prompt the person to put utensils down, or put your hand over theirs, if they are cramming food, so they chew/swallow every few mouthfuls
- Give a softer and more moist diet

Ensure a more calming environment, eg, reduce noise, use calming music

Serve courses separately, or even each course in a few smaller servings, giving a break between each, to ensure food is chewed, swallowed and cleared

If there has been a recent change in mood or behaviour, consult Chapter 3, questions 10 and 11, and seek medical advice if you are concerned

Too slow

Serve each course separately to retain heat and keep appetising

Use heat-retaining plate

Record dietary intake

Weigh the person regularly

Ensure food is high in calories, if only small amounts of diet are taken

Consider giving snacks in between meals

Tick if needed	2 MENTAL STATE AND BEHAVIOUR (continued)
	2(f) **(continued)** If difficulties are severe and the person is unable to maintain their nutritional status, they may need to be fed part or all of their meal Refer to the dietitian
	2(g) **Do they eat non-food items?** Ensure all involved are aware of this (including visitors) Lock away all harmful substances, eg, cleaning products, etc

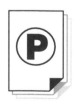

Feeding & Swallowing Disorders in Dementia © Jackie Kindell 2002 You may photocopy this page for instructional use only

Tick if needed	3 FEEDING SITUATION AND SKILLS
	3(a) Is the level of mealtime supervision inadequate? Time should be available for physical/verbal prompting as well as feeding Staff timetables in care homes/wards should take account of this need Inform management, so they are aware of the need regarding staffing levels Ensure staff are aware of the need for prompting Involve relatives or volunteers at mealtimes
	3(b) Is there a problem with the person's position when eating? Are they not fully upright, or is the table or chair not the correct height? Ensure the person is as upright as possible, eg, consider the type of chair and supports such as pillows, etc Avoid feeding in bed if possible – better to mobilise them to a chair Adjust their wheelchair, use a wheelchair tray, or transfer them to an appropriate chair, to ensure correct chair/table height Refer to the physiotherapist for advice on positioning/seating
	3(c) Does the person have difficulty self-feeding, for example, using or locating utensils or crockery on the table? Consider possible strategies for this: ◆ Cut food up (avoid doing this in front of them, so they don't feel like a child) ◆ Use a plate guard and a non-slip mat ◆ Give them only a fork or a spoon ◆ Put utensil directly into person's hand

Tick if needed	3 FEEDING SITUATION AND SKILLS (continued)
	3(c) **(continued)**
	Simplify the table – remove any unnecessary cutlery/crockery; serve one course at a time
	Use a plain tablecloth
	Ensure there is enough space on the table between people
	Consider use of finger foods for those who have difficulty using utensils
	Consider if larger-handled cutlery would be better
	Provide verbal and physical prompts, eg, putting the utensil back in the person's hand if they lose track of what they are doing during the meal
	As a last resort only, consider feeding them part or all of the meal if difficulties are severe
	Note: Remember many will still be able to hold a cup after the ability to use a fork or spoon has been lost, and this should be encouraged
	Refer to Occupational Therapy for advice about feeding management
	3(d) **Does the person eat or drink from other people's plates or glasses?**
	Increase the space between people, so individual boundaries are clearer
	Use physical or verbal prompts to help the person identify their food and utensils
	Supervision will be needed at mealtimes

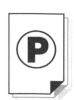

Tick if needed	3 FEEDING SITUATION AND SKILLS (continued)
	3(e) **Is the person distracted by other utensils or items on the table?** Simplify the mealtime environment: ◆ Serve one course at a time ◆ Put out only the cutlery and crockery that is needed ◆ Offer the person salt and sauce, and then remove it ◆ Show and explain the menu, and then remove it
	3(f) **Is the person messy when eating?** Improve positioning ◆ Move closer to the table ◆ Ensure they are upright Consider the advice in 3(c) for feeding difficulties Use napkins on their front and lap If nutritional intake is poor: ◆ Increase the calorie value of meals ◆ Give snacks in between meals ◆ Feed the person all or part of the meal as a last resort
	3(g) **Does the person mix different courses together?** Serve courses separately Do not point this out to the person, it is unlikely to help them in the future

Tick if needed	**3 FEEDING SITUATION AND SKILLS (continued)**
	3(h) **For those fed by another, are there any concerns regarding the feeder's approach?**
	Give advice outlining feeding approach as a collaborative effort, consider:
	◆ Sit facing the person, or slightly to their good side, if visual neglect is present
	◆ Make eye contact
	◆ Assist them, do not force
	◆ Use a gentle tone of voice
	◆ Use a calm approach, never rush the person
	◆ Give encouragement, tell the person about their food
	◆ Give verbal and nonverbal prompts to chew and swallow
	◆ Make allowance for any visual or hearing difficulties (see Section 1)
	◆ Use touch to encourage the person
	◆ Watch closely for each swallow, and only then give them another mouthful
	As far as possible, assign consistent staff member(s) to feed each person
	Consider involving close relatives to help with feeding, and provide advice or training for them

Tick if needed	4 ISSUES RELATED TO FOOD, DRINK, AND SWALLOWING
	4(a) Does the person experience significant drooling of saliva or food? Examine if change in food/fluid texture reduces drooling of food Improve posture Check if feeding technique could be improved Check the side effects of medication
	4(b) Are there any observable signs of tongue weakness or dysfunction, before or during eating? Examine the effects of consistency on this, and alter as necessary Experiment with different tastes, temperatures, size of bolus to increase sensation Check the side effects of medication
	4(c) Does the person have difficulty eating/swallowing particular consistencies? Difficulties should be clearly noted in their care plan, and this should be communicated to all staff and relatives **Problems with solids?** Give a softer and more moist diet (one that can be mashed with a fork), and avoid hard or fibrous foods that need a lot of chewing Use gravy or sauces (thickened appropriately) to soften food Encourage the person, wherever possible, to feed/partially feed themselves Try verbal prompts to chew and swallow, or indirect cues eg, 'that tastes nice'.

Tick if needed	**4 ISSUES RELATED TO FOOD, DRINK, AND SWALLOWING (continued)**
	4(c) (continued)
	Problems with bitty or lumpy food?
	Avoid bitty foods and foods with mixed textures, eg, crumbly biscuits, soup with bits, cereals with cold milk, food with skins or pips, etc
	Ensure food is soft in consistency throughout, eg, although food may be textured it should be soft enough to be able to be mashed with a fork
	If difficulties are severe, then smooth consistencies may be needed, but if food is puréed, each element should be puréed separately
	Problems with fluids?
	Try using a thickening agent in drinks; monitor if this reduces coughing/drooling
	If this is successful, ensure all staff are aware of this, and the correct consistency to mix and give
	Ensure this information has also been given to visitors, who may not appreciate the need for thickeners
	For all textures:
	Experiment with different tastes and temperatures, eg, sweet/sour, cold/hot
	Set a date to review dietary changes, or a method for staff to review progress and contact you for further advice/review, etc
	4(d) **Is there a delay in triggering the swallow?**
	Consider altering the consistency of food/fluid:
	◆ Are they at risk on thin fluids?
	◆ Would softer/more moist food be better?

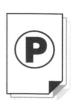

Tick if needed	4 ISSUES RELATED TO FOOD, DRINK, AND SWALLOWING (continued)
	4(d) **(continued)**
	Try verbal prompts to swallow, or indirect cues eg, 'this tastes nice'
	Wait, and then examine if carefully giving the next mouthful helps trigger the event
	Involve the person as much as possible in holding the cup or spoon, etc
	4(e) **Is there repeated coughing, throat clearing or choking after swallowing?**
	Consider the effects of consistency on this, and alter as necessary
	Examine if improving posture reduces this
	Examine if feeding style or rate is exacerbating this
	If difficulties are severe, see 5(b)
	4(f) **Is there a change to a wet, gargly voice quality after swallowing?**
	Consider if this could be a sign of silent aspiration
	Note the effects of consistency on this, and alter texture as necessary, eg, would thickened fluids be helpful?
	Improve posture
	Examine if feeding style or rate is exacerbating this
	4(g) **Does the person need several swallows to clear each mouthful?**
	Advise staff about the signs to observe, and the need for a slower feeding rate
	Note the effects of consistency on this, and alter texture as necessary eg, if softer and more moist food would help

Tick if needed	4 ISSUES RELATED TO FOOD, DRINK, AND SWALLOWING (continued)
	4(h) **Does the person have difficulty with particular foods, eg, bread or meat, or with swallowing tablets?** List these clearly in their care plan, so they can be avoided Consult with pharmacy if tablets can be crushed, or available in syrup/liquid form
	4(i) **Is the size of mouthfuls taken a concern?** **Too large** Cut all food into small pieces before presenting it Encourage the person to take smaller mouthfuls, and eat at a slower rate If also cramming, prompt to put down utensils and chew/swallow every few mouthfuls, or put your hand over theirs to physically prompt them Give them a softer and more moist diet if coughing or choking occurs **Too small** Verbally encourage the person to take large mouthfuls Give smaller, but more regular meals Give snacks in between meals Look for signs of depression (see Chapter 3, question 10)
	4(j) **Is the temperature of the food or drink too hot, or too cold?** Ensure the temperature of all food and drink is appropriate Serve courses separately, to keep them appetising Use insulated or heat-retaining plate for slow eaters Consider advice in 2(e) for slow eaters

Tick if needed	4 ISSUES RELATED TO FOOD, DRINK, AND SWALLOWING (continued)
	4(k) Does the person leave a large proportion of their meal?
	Advise staff to keep a record of dietary intake and weight
	Give smaller but more regular meals
	Give snacks in between meals
	Increase calorie value of meals and/or use supplements
	Consider if this is variable and why eg, due to time of day, fatigue, taste, or possible effects of medication (see 2(e) for advice on food refusals)
	Refer to dietitian for advice
	4(l) Does the person have any food and drink preferences or dislikes?
	List the person's religious/cultural/personal needs with regard to food (eg, ask relatives for this information)
	Current likes and dislikes should be clearly listed in their care plan
	Accommodate likes into present textures/diet if possible eg, if they previously liked chocolate, try chocolate mousse
	Be aware that habits may change as the dementia progresses
	Note especially increased consumption of sweet foods
	4(m) Is food left in the person's mouth or cheeks at the end of a meal?
	Recommend mouth care after each meal
	Advise that the person does not lie down immediately after eating

Tick if needed	**5 SEVERE SWALLOWING PROBLEMS**
	5(a) **Is further investigation of their swallowing required, eg, videofluoroscopy?** Consider: ◆ If with time and prompting, will the person be able to cooperate with this? ◆ Will this provide additional useful information, or alter management?
	5(b) **Does the person have severe swallowing problems across all textures?** If tube-feeding is to be considered, the following areas should be highlighted: 1 What is the aim, or benefit, of tube-feeding? 2 What are the burdens, or drawbacks, of tube-feeding? 3 Are they to be kept totally nil by mouth if they are to be tube-fed? 4 Is the person competent to take this decision? 5 If they are not competent, then in English law, their doctor can decide if treatment can be provided without consent, by considering what is in their 'best interests', following consultation with the family and multi-disciplinary team. Check for guidelines in your country/state regarding this. 6 If tube-feeding is to be initiated, then what goals have been set to measure effectiveness? 7 Has a review date been set to examine these goals? 8 If tube-feeding is not initiated, then is a clear management plan outlined to manage eating, drinking and overall comfort? 9 Have goals been set to manage the effectiveness of this plan? 10 Has a review date been set to examine these goals? 11 Have the person and their relatives been given adequate information and support, and been involved in discussions? 12 Have the effects on staff been considered and managed appropriately?

Bibliography

Ackerman TF, 1996, 'The Moral Implications of Medical Uncertainty: Tube Feeding Demented Patients', *Journal of the American Geriatrics Society* 44, pp1265–7.

Allen NHP & Burns A, 1995, 'The Non-Cognitive Features of Dementia', *Reviews in Clinical Gerontology* 5, pp57–75.

Alzheimer's Society, 2000, *Food for Thought*, Survey by the Alzheimer's Society, London.

Athlin E & Norberg A, 1987a, 'Caregivers Attitudes to and Interpretations of the Behaviour of Severely Demented Patients During Feeding in a Patient Assignment Care System', *International Journal of Nursing Studies* 24, pp145–53.

Athlin E & Norberg A, 1987b, 'Interactions Between the Severely Demented Patient and his Caregiver During Feeding', *Scandinavian Journal of Caring Science* 1, pp117–23.

Athlin E & Norberg A, 1998, 'Interaction Between Patients with Severe Dementia and Their Caregivers During Feeding in a Task-Assignment Versus a Patient-Assignment Care System', *European Nurse* 3(4), pp215–27.

Barer DH, 1989, 'The Natural History and Functional Consequences of Dysphagia after Hemispheric Stroke', *Journal of Neurology, Neurosurgery and Psychiatry* 52, pp236–41.

Basavaraju NG, Silverstone FA, Libow LS & Paraskevas K, 1981, 'Primitive Reflexes and Perceptual Sensory Tests in the Elderly and their Usefulness in Dementia', *Journal of Chronic Diseases* 34, pp367–77.

Batchelor B, Neilsen S, & Sexton K, 1996, 'Issues in Maintaining Hydration in Nursing Home Patients Who Aspirate Thin Liquids', *Journal of Medical Speech-Language Pathology* 4(3), pp217–21.

Bathgate D, Snowden J, Varma A, Blackshaw A & Neary D, (2001) 'Behaviour in Frontemporal Dementia, Alzheimer's Disease and Vascular Dementia', *Acta Neurologica Scandinavica* 103, pp1–13.

Bayles K, 1995, 'Communication Assessment – Interventions and the Future', presentation given 11 July 1995, Wolfson Centre, London.

Bazemore PH, Tonkonogy J & Ananth R, 1991, 'Dysphagia in Psychiatric Patients: Clinical and Videofluoroscopic Study', *Dysphagia* 6, pp2–5.

Beck C, 1981, 'Dining Experience of the Institutionalised Elderly', *Journal of Gerontological Nursing* 7, pp104–7.

Blandford G, Watkins L, Mulvihill B & Taylor B, 1998, 'Assessing Abnormal Feeding Behaviour in Dementia: A Taxonomy and Initial Findings', *Weight Loss and Eating Behaviour in Alzheimer's Patients, Research and Practice in Alzheimer's Disease*, Springer Publishing.

British Association for Parenteral and Enteral Nutrition, 1999, 'Ethical and Legal Aspects of Clinical Hydration and Nutritional Support', *A Report for BAPEN by JE Lennard-Jones*.

British Medical Association, 1999, *Withholding and Withdrawing Life-prolonging Medical Treatment, guidance for decision making*, British Medical Journal Books.

British National Formulary, 2000, British Medical Association, London & Royal Pharmaceutical Society of Great Britain, London.

Burge P, 1994, 'Textured Soft Diets and Feeding Techniques Among the Elderly Mentally Ill', *Journal of Human Nutrition and Dietetics* 7, pp191–8.

Burns A, Howard R & Pettit W, 1995, *Alzheimer's disease: a medical companion*, Blackwell Scientific.

Burton-Jones J, 1998, 'Sharing the Experience of Mealtimes in Homes', *Dementia Care* 13, p9.

Carlsson G, 1984, 'Masticatory Efficiency: The Effect of Age, the Loss of Teeth and Prosthetic Rehabilitation', *International Dental Journal* 34, pp98–104.

Caroline Walker Trust, The, 1995, 'Eating Well for Older People. Practical and Nutritional Guidelines for Food in Residential and Nursing Homes and for Community Meals. Report of an Expert Working Group', The Caroline Walker Trust, London.

Cherney LR, 1994, *'Clinical Management of Dysphagia in Adults and Children'*, 2nd Edn, Aspen Publications.

Cookson J, Crammer J & Heine B, 1993, *'The Use of Drugs in Psychiatry'*, 4th Edn, Gaskell.

Coyne ML & Hoskins L, 1997, 'Improving Eating Behaviours in Dementia Using Behavioural Strategies', *Clinical Nursing Research* 6(3) August, pp275–90.

Cullen P, Abid F, Patel A, Coope B & Ballard CG, 1997, 'Eating Disorders in Dementia', *International Journal of Geriatric Psychiatry* 12, pp559–62.

Davies AD & Snaith PA, 1980, 'The Social Behaviour of Geriatric Patients at Mealtimes: An Observational and an Intervention Study', *Age and Aging* 9, pp93–9.

Denney A, 1997, 'Quiet Music – An Intervention for Mealtime Agitation', *Journal of Gerontological Nursing* July, pp16–23.

Du W, DiLuca C & Growdon JH, 1993, 'Weight loss in Alzheimer's Disease', *Journal of Geriatric Psychiatry and Neurology* 6, pp34–8.

Eaton M, Mitchell-Bonair IL & Friedmann E, 1986, 'The Effect of Touch on Nutritional Intake of Chronic Organic Brain Syndrome Patients', *Journal of Gerontology* 41(5), pp 611–16.

Ek AC, Larsson J, von Schenck H, Thorslund S, Unosson M & Bjurulf P, 1990, 'The Correlation Between Energy, Malnutrition and Clinical Outcome in Elderly Hospital Population', *Clinical Nutrition* 9, pp185–9.

Ekberg O & Feinberg MJ, 1991, 'Altered Swallowing Function in Elderly Patients without Dysphagia: Radiologic Findings in 56 Cases', *American Journal of Radiology* 156, pp1181–4.

Feinberg MJ, Ekberg O, Segall L & Tully J, 1992, 'Deglutition in Elderly Patients with Dementia: Findings of Videofluorographic Evaluation and Impact on Staging and Management', *Radiology* 183(3), pp811–14.

Finucane TE & Bynum JPW, 1996, 'Use of Tube Feeding to Prevent Aspiration Pneumonia', *Lancet* 348, pp1421–4.

Finucane TE, Christmas C and Travis K, 1999, 'Tube Feeding in Patients with Advanced Dementia, *JAMA*, 282(14), pp1365–70.

Ford G, 1996, 'Putting Feeding Back into the Hands of Patients', *Journal of Psychosocial Nursing* 34(5), pp35–9.

Gillick MR, 2000, 'Rethinking the Role of Tube Feeding in Patients with Advanced Dementia', *The New England Journal of Medicine*, 20 Jan, pp206–10.

Goldberg D, Benjamin S & Creed F, 1987, *Psychiatry in Medical Practice*, Tavistock Publications, London and New York.

Grimes AM, 1995, 'Auditory changes', Lubinski R (ed), *Dementia and Communication*, Singular Publishing Co.

Groher ME & Bukatman R, 1986, 'The Prevalence of Swallowing Disorders in Two Teaching Hospitals', *Dysphagia* 1, pp3–6.

Groher ME, 1990, 'Ethical Dilemmas in Providing Nutrition', *Dysphagia* 5, pp102–9.

Groher ME, 1997, *'Dysphagia, Diagnosis and Management'* 3rd Edn, Butterworth-Heinemann.

Guyonnet S, Nourhashemi F, Ousset PJ, Micas M, Ghisolfi A, Vellas B & Albarede JL, 1998, 'Factors Associated with Weight Loss in Alzheimer's Disease', *Weight Loss and Eating Behaviour in Alzheimer's Patients, Research and Practice in Alzheimer's Disease*, Springer Publishing.

Hart S & Semple JM, 1990, '*Neuropsychology and the Dementias*, Taylor & Francis.

Horner J, Massey MD, Riski JE, Lathrop MA & Chase KN, 1988, 'Aspiration Following Stroke: Clinical Correlates and Outcome, *Neurology* 38, pp1359–62.

Hudson HM, Daubert CR & Mills RH, 2000, 'The Interdependency of Protein-Energy Malnutrition, Aging, and Dysphagia', *Dysphagia* 15, pp31–8.

International Classification of Diseases, World Health Organisation, 1992, Tenth Revisions of the International Classification of Diseases and Related Health Problems. Clinical descriptions and diagnostic guidelines', World Health Organisation.

Kayser-Jones J & Schell E, 1997, 'The Mealtime Experience of a Cognitively Impaired Elder: Ineffective and Effective Strategies', *Journal of Gerontological Nursing* July, pp33–9.

Keene J & Hope T, 1998, 'Natural History of Hyperphagia and Other Eating Changes in Dementia', *International Journal of Geriatric Psychiatry* 13, pp700–6.

Kline N & Sexton DL, 1996, 'Eating Behaviors of Nursing Home Residents Who Display Agitation', *Nursing Management*, November.

Kolodny V & Malek A, 1991, ' Improving Feeding Skills', *Journal of Gerontological Nursing* 17(6), pp20–4.

Larsson J, Unosson M, Ek AC, Nilsson L, Thorsland S & Bjurulf P, 1990, 'Effects of Dietary Supplement in 501 Geriatric Patients – A Randomised Study', *Clinical Nutrition* 9, pp179–84.

LeClerc CM & Wells DL, 1998, 'Use of a Content Methodology Process to Enhance Feeding Abilities Threatened by Ideational Apraxia in People with Alzheimer's-type Dementia', *Geriatric Nursing* 19(5), pp261–8.

Leeds M, 1960, 'Senile Recession: A Clinical Entity?' *Journal of the American Geriatrics Society* 8, pp122–31

Lennard-Jones JE, 1999, 'Ethical and Legal Aspects of Clinical Hydration and Nutritional Support: A Report for The British Association for Parenteral and Enteral Nutrition'.

Lieberman AN, Horowitz L, Redmond P, Pachter L, Lieberman I & Leibowitz M, 1980, 'Dysphagia in Parkinson's Disease', *American Journal of Gastroenterology* 74(2), pp157–60.

Logemann J, 1983, *Evaluation and Treatment of Swallowing Disorders*, College Hill Press.

Logemann J, 1998, *Evaluation and Treatment of Swallowing Disorders*, 2nd Edn, College Hill Press.

Logemann J, 2000, *Advanced Dysphagia Course, Great Britain.*

Logemann JA, Pauloski B, Colangelo L, Lazarus C, Fujiu M & Kahrilas PJ, 1995, 'Effects of a Sour Bolus on Oropharyngeal Swallowing Measures in Patients with Neurogenic Dysphagia', *Journal of Speech and Hearing Research* 38, pp556–63.

Malone N, 1994, 'Hydration in the Terminally Ill Patient', *Nursing Standard* 8(43), pp29–32.

Mann DMA, Neary D & Testa H, 1994, *Colour Atlas and Text of Adult Dementias*, Mosby-Wolfe Publishing.

Martin P, 1987, *'Care of the Mentally Ill'*, Macmillan Education.

Mckeith IG, Galasko D, Kosaka K, Perry EK, Dickson DW, Hansen LA, Salmon DP, Lowe J, Mirra SS, Byrne EJ, Lennox G, Quinn NP, Edwardson JA, Ince PG, Bergeron C, Burns A, Miller BL, Lovestone S, Collerton D, Jansen ENH, Ballard C, de Vos RAI, Wilcock DM, Jellinger KA & Perry RH, 1996, 'Consensus guidelines for the clinical and pathological diagnosis of dementia with Lewy bodies (DLB): Report of the consortium of DLB international workshop', *Neurology* 47, pp1113–24.

Melin I & Gotestam KG, 1981, 'The Effects of Rearranging Ward Routines on Communication and Eating Behaviours of Psychogeriatric Patients', *Journal of Applied Behaviour Analysis* 14, pp47–51.

Miller BL, Darby AL, Swartz JR, Yener GG & Mena I, 1995, 'Dietary Changes, Compulsions and Sexual Behaviour in Frontotemporal Degeneration', *Dementia* 6(4), pp195–9.

Miskovitz P, Weg A & Groher M, 1988, 'Must Dysphagic Patients Always Receive Food and Water?' *Dysphagia* 2, pp125–6.

Mitchell SL, Kiely DK & Lipsitz LA, 1997, 'The Risk Factors and Impact on Survival of Feeding Tube Placement in Nursing Home Residents with Severe Cognitive Impairment', *Archives in International Medicine* 157(10), pp327–32.

Morris CH, Hope RA & Fairburn CG, 1989, 'Eating Habits in Dementia', *British Journal of Psychiatry* 154, pp801–6.

Mungas D, Cooper JK, Weiler PG, Gietzen D, Franzi C & Bernick C, 1990, 'Dietary Preference for Sweet Foods in Patients with Dementia', *Journal of The American Geriatrics Society* 38, pp999–1007.

National Conference of Catholic Bishops, 1995, *Ethical and Religious Directives for Catholic Health Care Services*, Washington DC, US, Catholic Conference.

Neary D, 1999, 'Classification of the Dementias', *Reviews in Clinical Gerontology* 9, pp55–64.

Neary D, Snowden JS, Gustafson L, Passant U, Stuss D, Black S, Freedman M, Kertesz A, Roberts PH, Albert M, Boone K, Miller BL, Cummings J & Benson DF, 1998, 'Frontotemporal Lobar Degeneration: A Consensus on Clinical Diagnostic Criteria', *Neurology* 51(December), pp1546–54.

Nilsson H, Ekberg O, Olsson R & Hindfelt B, 'Quantitative Aspects of Swallowing in an Elderly Nondysphagic Population', *Dysphagia* 11, pp180–4.

Norberg A, Norberg B, Gippert H & Bexell G, 1980, 'Ethical Conflicts in Long Term Care of the Aged: Nutritional Problems and the Patient-Care Worker Relationship, *British Medical Journal* 280, pp377–9.

Osborn CL & Marshall MJ, 1993, 'Self-Feeding Performance in Nursing Home Residents', *Journal of Gerontological Nursing* 19(3), pp7–14.

Peck A, Cohen CE & Mulvihill MN, 1990, 'Long-Term Enteral Feeding of Aged Demented Nursing Home Patients', *Journal of the American Geriatrics Society* 38, pp1195–8.

Priefer BA & Robbins J, 1997, 'Eating Changes in Mild-Stage Alzheimer's Disease: A Pilot Study, *Dysphagia* 12, pp212–21.

Purandare N, Allen NHP & Burns A, 2000, 'Behavioural and Psychological Symptoms of Dementia', *Reviews in Clinical Gerontology* 10, pp245–60.

Ragneskog H, Brane G, Karlsson I & Kihlgren M, 1996, 'Influence of Dinner Music on Food Intake and Symptoms in Dementia', *Scandinavian Journal of Caring Science* 10(1), pp11–17.

Relatives Association (Great Britain), The, 1995, *'Dental Care for Older People in Homes'*, The Relatives Association, London.

Rosin AJ, Sonnenblick M, 1998, 'Autonomy and Paternalism in Geriatric Medicine: the Jewish Ethical Approach to Issues of Feeding Terminally Ill Patients, and to Cardiopulmonary Resuscitation', *Journal of Medical Ethics* 24, pp44–8.

Rudmand D & Feller AG, 'Protein Calorie Under-Nutrition in the Nursing Home Patient', *Journal of the American Geriatrics Society* 37, pp173–83.

Sandman P, Adolfsson R, Nygren C, Hallmans G & Winblad B, 1987, 'Nutritional Status and Dietary Intake in Institutionalised Patients with Alzheimer's Disease and Multi-Infarct Dementia', *Journal of the American Geriatrics Society* 35, pp31–8.

Schiffman SS & Graham BG, 2000, 'Taste and Smell Perception Affect Appetite and Immunity in the Elderly', *European Journal of Clinical Nutrition* 54(3), pp54–63.

Schostak RZ, 1994, 'Jewish Ethical Guidelines for Resuscitation and Artificial Nutrition and Hydration of the Dying Elderly', *Journal of Medical Ethics* 20, pp93–100.

Serradura-Russell A, 1992, 'Ethical Dilemmas in Dysphagia Management and the Right to a Natural Death', *Dysphagia* 7, pp102–5.

Sheiman SL, 1996, 'Tube Feeding the Demented Nursing Home Resident', *Journal of the American Geriatrics Society* 44(10).

Sheth N & Diner WC, 1988, 'Swallowing Problems in the Elderly', *Dysphagia* 2, pp209–15.

Sidenvall B & Ek AC, 1993, 'Long-Term Care Patients and their Dietary Intake Related to Eating Ability and Nutritional Needs: Nursing Staff Interventions', *Journal of Advanced Nursing* 18, pp565–73.

Siebens H, Trupe E, Siebens A, Cook F, Anshen S, Hanauer R & Oster G, 1986, 'Correlates and Consequences of Eating Dependency in Institutionalized Elderly', *Journal of the American Geriatrics Society*, 34(3).

Singh S, Mulley GP & Losowsky MS, 1988, 'Why are Alzheimer's Patients Thin?', *Age and Ageing* 17, pp21–9.

Smith J & Shieham A, 1979, 'How Dental Conditions Handicap the Elderly', *Community Dent Oral Epidemiology* 7, pp305–10.

Snowden JS, 1999, 'Contribution to the Differential Diagnosis of Dementias 1: Neuropsychology, *Reviews in Clinical Gerontology* 9, pp65–72.

Sokoloff LG & Pavlakovic R, 1997, 'Neuroleptic-Induced Dysphagia', *Dysphagia* 12, pp177–9.

Spencer B, Pritchard-Howarth M, Lee T & Jack C, 2000, 'Won't drink? Can't drink', *Age and Ageing* 29(2), p185.

Steele CM, Greenwood C, Robertson C & Seidman-Carlson R, 1997, 'Mealtime Difficulties in a Home for the Aged: Not just Dysphagia', *Dysphagia* 12, pp43–50.

Stoschus B & Allescher HD, 1993, 'Drug-Induced Dysphagia', *Dysphagia* 8, pp154–9.

Suski NS & Nielson CC, 1989, 'Factors Affecting Food Intake in Women with Alzheimer's Type Dementia in Long Term Care', *Journal of the American Dietetics Association* 89, pp1770–3.

Tracey JF, Logemann JA, Kahrilas PJ, Jacob P, Kobara M & Krugler C, 1989, 'Preliminary Observations on the Effects of Age on Oropharyngeal Deglutition', *Dysphagia* 4, pp90–4.

Trinkle DB, Burns A, Levy R, 1992, 'Abnormal Eating Behaviour in Dementia: a descriptive study', *International Journal of Geriatric Psychiatry* 7, pp799–803.

VOICES, 1998, *'Eating Well for Older People with Dementia'*, Voluntary Organisations Involved in Caring in the Elderly Sector, Beechwood House, Wyllotts Close, Potters Bar, Herts, EN6 2HN (tel 01707 651777).

Volicer L, 1998, 'Tube Feeding in Alzheimer's Disease is Avoidable', Weight Loss and Eating Behaviour in Alzheimers's Disease, *Research and Practice in Alzheimer's Disease*, pp71–4.

Volicer L, Seltzer B, Rheaumme Y, Fabiszewski K, Hertz L, Shapiro R & Innis P, 1987, 'Progression of Alzheimer Type Dementia in Institutionalised Patients: A Cross Sectional Study', *Journal of Applied Gerontology* 6, pp83–94.

Volicer L, Seltzer MD, Rheaume Y, Karner J, Glennon M, Riley ME & Crino P, 1989, 'Eating Difficulties in Patients with Probable Dementia of the Alzheimer's Type', *Journal of Geriatric Psychiatry and Neurology* 2(4), pp188–95.

Volicer L, Rheaume Y & Cyr D, 1994, 'Treatment of Depression in Advanced Alzheimer's Disease Using Sertraline', *Journal of Geriatric Psychiatry and Neurology* 7, pp227–9.

Walls AWG, Cooper I, Steele JG, Finch J, Smithers G, Wenlock RW & Clarke PC, 1997, 'National Diet and Nutrition Survey: People Aged 65 Years or Over. Volume 2: Report of the Dental Survey', The Stationery Office, London.

Wang S, Fukagawa N, Hossain M & Ooi W, 1998, 'Longitudinal Weight Changes, Length of Survival and Energy Requirements of Long Term Care Residents with Dementia', *Weight Loss and Eating Behaviour in Alzheimer's Patients, Research and Practice in Alzheimer's Disease*, Springer Publishing.

Watson R, 1997, 'Undernutrition, Weight Loss and Feeding Difficulty in Elderly Patients with Dementia: a nursing perspective', *Reviews in Clinical Gerontology* 7, pp317–26.

Watson R, 1993, 'Measuring Feeding Difficulty in Patients with Dementia: Perspectives and Problems', *Journal of Advanced Nursing* 18, pp25–32.

Zimmer JG, 1975, 'Characteristics of Patients and Care Provided in Health-related and Skilled Nursing Facilities', *Med Care* 13, pp992–1010.

Titles of related interest from Speechmark

Working with Dysphagia

Lizzy Marks & Deirdre Rainbow

The caseloads of speech & language therapists have increasingly included work with dysphagia clients. This timely and practical text will be of enormous comfort to all clinicians working with dysphagia and is suitable for those involved in a range of settings and a diversity of client groups including those with acquired neurological disorders and learning difficulties. With its perspective on current everyday practice, this accessible and highly practical volume fills a gap in an area where practical and workable material is much sought after.

Among areas covered are anatomy and physiology, theories of normal & impaired swallow, respiration & aspiration and a discussion of multidisciplinary working as well as legal, health & safety and ethical issues.

Contents include
The normal swallow; Respiration & aspiration; Introduction to assessment; Subjective assessment; Objective assessment; General issues in management; Oral stage management; Pharyngeal stage management; Tracheotomies & ventilators; Nutrition & hydration; Legal & professional issues; Health & safety; Making ethical decisions; Training other professionals.

The Essential Dementia Care Handbook
A Good Practice Guide

Edited by Graham Stokes & Fiona Goudie

This new title replaces the successful *Working with Dementia*, which has been a vital handbook for many years for all those working with this group of clients. This long-awaited edition captures the essence of what has happened over the past decade in dementia care. It draws together many new ideas and practical approaches from a wide variety of professionals working at the leading edge of the provision of services to people with dementia. It can be read in its entirety as a comprehensive account of current best practice, but the chapters are designed to stand alone. This essential handbook will replace *Working with Dementia* as the pocket 'bible' for all care staff.

- Beginning with the diagnosis of dementia and other problems associated with ageing, this book considers assessment, the person-centred model of dementia, rehabilitation and therapy.

- The contributors draw on their considerable and varied experiences to outline practical interventions,

illustrating their ideas by case studies which provide a stimulating insight into contemporary understanding and practice.

- Nursing staff, occupational therapists, residential care workers, social workers and all those in day-to-day contact with elderly people will be inspired by this entirely new edition.

Contents include
Dementia: causes & neuropsychology; Cognitive & behavioural assessment; Person-centred approaches to understanding; Memory clinics; Activity, occupation & stimulation; Challenging behaviour; Depression & distress; Therapeutic relationships; Medication; Carers & caring.

Challenging Behaviour in Dementia
A Person-Centred Approach

Graham Stokes

Understanding socially disruptive behaviour in dementia is never easy and treatment is often characterised by policies of control and containment. This book, which is the result of Graham Stokes' 15 years of clinical work with people who are challenging:

- Disputes the traditional medical model of dementia and asserts that if we reach behind the barrier of cognitive devastation and decipher the cryptic messages, it can be shown that much behaviour is not meaningless but meaningful;

- Contrasts the medical interpretation that sees anti-social behaviour as mere symptoms of disease with a person-centred interpretation that resonates change and resolution;

- Offers a radical and innovative interpretation of challenging behaviour consistent with the new culture of dementia care, focusing on needs to be met rather than problems to be managed.

Contents include
Dementia: No Longer a 'Silent Epidemic'; Assessment of Behaviour in Dementia; The 'Medical Disease' Model of Dementia; A Person with Dementia; The Environmental Context of Dementia; The Needs of People with Dementia; Taxonomies of Possible Explanations; Behavioural, Ecobehavioural and Functional Analysis; Resolution Therapy; Resolution: Needs to be Met, not Problems to be Managed; Working with Unmet Need; The Challenge of Confusion

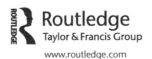
Routledge
Taylor & Francis Group
www.routledge.com